AF510923

Handbook on Cerebral Venous Thrombosis

Frontiers of Neurology and Neuroscience

Vol. 23

Series Editor

J. Bogousslavsky, Montreux

Handbook on Cerebral Venous Thrombosis

Volume Editors

V. Caso, Perugia
G. Agnelli, Perugia
M. Paciaroni, Perugia

24 figures, 2 in color, and 21 tables, 2008

KARGER

Basel · Freiburg · Paris · London · New York ·
Bangalore · Bangkok · Singapore · Tokyo · Sydney

Dr. Valeria Caso, MD, PhD
Prof. Giancarlo Agnelli, MD
Dr. Maurizio Paciaroni
Stroke Unit and Division of Cardiovascular Medicine
Department of Internal Medicine, University of Perugia
Santa Maria della Misericordia Hospital
Via Dottori
Sant' Andrea delle Fratte
IT–06126 Perugia

Library of Congress Cataloging-in-Publication Data

Handbook on cerebral venous thrombosis / volume editors, V. Caso, G. Agnelli, M. Paciaroni.
p. ; cm. – (Frontiers of neurology and neuroscience, ISSN 1660–4431 ; v. 23)
Includes bibliographical references and indexes.
ISBN 978–3–8055–8378–7 (hard cover : alk. paper)
1. Sinus thrombosis. I. Caso, V. (Valeria) II. Agnelli, Giancarlo. III. Paciaroni, M. (Maurizio) IV. Series.
[DNLM: 1. Intracranial Thrombosis–diagnosis. 2. Intracranial Thrombosis–radiotherapy. 3. Sinus Thrombosis, Intracranial–diagnosis. 4. Sinus Thrombosis, Intracranial–radiotherapy. WL 355 H2367 2008]
RC388.5.H3453 2008
616.8′1075–dc22
2007037850

Bibliographic Indices. This publication is listed in bibliographic services, including Current Contents® and Index Medicus.

Disclaimer. The statements, options and data contained in this publication are solely those of the individual authors and contributors and not of the publisher and the editor(s). The appearance of advertisements in the book is not a warranty, endorsement, or approval of the products or services advertised or of their effectiveness, quality or safety. The publisher and the editor(s) disclaim responsibility for any injury to persons or property resulting from any ideas, methods, instructions or products referred to in the content or advertisements.

Drug Dosage. The authors and the publisher have exerted every effort to ensure that drug selection and dosage set forth in this text are in accord with current recommendations and practice at the time of publication. However, in view of ongoing research, changes in government regulations, and the constant flow of information relating to drug therapy and drug reactions, the reader is urged to check the package insert for each drug for any change in indications and dosage and for added warnings and precautions. This is particularly important when the recommended agent is a new and/or infrequently employed drug.

All rights reserved. No part of this publication may be translated into other languages, reproduced or utilized in any form or by any means electronic or mechanical, including photocopying, recording, microcopying, or by any information storage and retrieval system, without permission in writing from the publisher.

© Copyright 2008 by S. Karger AG, P.O. Box, CH–4009 Basel (Switzerland)
www.karger.com
Printed in Switzerland on acid-free and non-aging paper (ISO 9706) by Reinhardt Druck, Basel
ISSN 1660–4431
ISBN 978–3–8055–8378–7

Contents

Caso V, Agnelli G, Paciaroni M (eds): Handbook on Cerebral Venous Thrombosis.
Front Neurol Neurosci. Basel, Karger, 2008, vol 23, pp 1–3

Introduction

L.J. Kappelle

University Department of Neurology, University Medical Center Utrecht,
Rudolph Magnus Institute for Neurosciences, Utrecht, The Netherlands

Cerebral veins contain about 70% of the total cerebral blood volume, but cerebral venous sinus thrombosis (CVST) occurs about thousand times less often than arterial stroke. Arterial and venous stroke cause different neurological deficits and occur in people of different ages. About half of the patients with an arterial stroke are older than 75 years, whereas CVST most often affects young adults and children. It is not a manifestation of atherosclerosis, but usually is associated with a prothrombotic state due to (inherited) thrombophilia, other blood disorders, dehydration, infectious diseases, cancer, or more rare causes. In about a quarter of the patients with CVST the cause remains unknown. The annual incidence is currently estimated to be 3–4 cases per 1 million people. Three out of 4 people with CVST are women. One out of 8 patients will die or remain handicapped as a result of CVST [1]. During the past decade, modern neuroimaging techniques have improved the diagnostic process and together with the increased awareness this will probably result in increased recognition in the future.

CVST has received far less attention in clinical research than arterial stroke. The small number of patients with CVST limits the performance of large epidemiological studies and clinical trials on a scale similar to that in patients with arterial stroke. The largest trial in the field of CVST counted only 60 patients [2]. So far, only three trials have been performed to study treatment with anticoagulation. All three trials showed a nonsignificant benefit of anticoagulant treatment as compared with placebo. A meta-analysis of these studies showed a nonsignificant reduction in the pooled relative risk of death or dependency of 0.46 (95% confidence interval: 0.16–1.31) [3].

Thanks to the efforts of Jose Ferro and his colleagues, the International Study on Cerebral Vein and Dural Sinus Thrombosis (ISCVT) was initiated [1]. This collaborative initiative has now resulted in several joint papers and has substantially increased our knowledge. However, information obtained from the ISCVT is based on observational data and international multicenter trials are still to be awaited. Not only a conclusive trial about the type and duration of anticoagulation therapy, but also large trials about the usefulness of corticosteroids or endovascular thrombolysis would add substantially to our knowledge on how to best treat patients with CVST.

Thrombosis of the cerebral veins may cause focal deficits due to local effects of venous obstruction, but also more generalized effects as a result of increased cerebrospinal fluid pressure caused by blocking of the major sinuses. In the majority of patients, these two processes occur simultaneously [4]. The course and clinical features of CVST are highly variable. It is only after the introduction of computerized tomography and (particularly) magnetic resonance imaging that verification of the diagnosis during life has become part of daily clinical practice and that, as a result, the clinical spectrum of the disease has enormously increased. It is now well known that the clinical features of CVST are extraordinarily variable. Consequently, the diagnosis may be difficult. The average delay from the onset of symptoms to the diagnosis is 7 days [1]. Patients may present to an ear, nose and throat surgeon with recurrent ear infections and headache, to a pediatrician with headache and vomiting, to an obstetrician because of a complicated pregnancy or puerperium, to an ophthalmologist because of blurred vision, to an internist because of vague symptoms in the context of a systemic disease, to a neurologist because of epileptic seizures, or to a neurosurgeon because of chronic intracranial hypertension. The variety of clinical features and the large number of specialists dealing with the care of patients with CVST have resulted in papers in peer-reviewed journals of many different disciplines, making a clear and concise overview difficult. For this reason, the current book edited by experts in the field of stroke from Perugia, Italy, that covers the full spectrum of CVST, should be welcomed as a useful clinical guide for all physicians who are involved in the care of patients with CVST.

References

1 Ferro JM, Canhao P, Stam J, Bousser MG, Barinagarrementeria F: Prognosis of cerebral vein and dural sinus thrombosis: results of the International Study on Cerebral Vein and Dural Sinus Thrombosis (ISCVT). Stroke 2004;35:664–670.

2 de Bruijn SFTM, Stam J: Randomized, placebo-controlled trial of anticoagulant treatment with low-molecular-weight heparin for cerebral sinus thrombosis. Stroke 1999;30:484–488.

3 Stam J, De Bruijn SFTM, DeVeber G: Anticoagulation for cerebral sinus thrombosis. Cochrane Database Syst Rev 2002;4:CD002005.

4 Stam J: Thrombosis of the cerebral veins and sinuses. N Engl J Med 2005;352:1791–1798.

Prof. L.J. Kappelle
University Department of Neurology, University Medical Center Utrecht
Rudolph Magnus Institute for Neurosciences
NL–3584 CX Utrecht (The Netherlands)
Tel. +31 30 250 7975, Fax +31 30 254 2100, E-Mail l.kappelle@neuro.azu.nl

Caso V, Agnelli G, Paciaroni M (eds): Handbook on Cerebral Venous Thrombosis.
Front Neurol Neurosci. Basel, Karger, 2008, vol 23, pp 4–15

Anatomy of Cerebral Veins and Sinuses

Türker Kılıç[a], *Akın Akakın*[b]

[a]Sections of Neurovascular and Neurooncological Surgery, [b]Department of Neurosurgery, Marmara University, Istanbul, Turkey

Abstract

The veins of the brain have no muscular tissue in their thin walls and possess no valves. They emerge from the brain and lie in the subarachnoid space. They pierce the arachnoid mater and the meningeal layer of the dura and drain into the cranial venous sinuses. The cerebral venous system can be divided into a superficial and a deep system. The superficial system comprises sagittal sinuses and cortical veins, which drain superficial surfaces of both cerebral hemispheres. The deep system consists of the lateral sinus, straight sinus and sigmoid sinus along with draining deeper cortical veins. Both of these systems mostly drain into internal jugular veins. Generally, venous blood drains into the nearest venous sinus or, in the case of blood draining from the deepest structures, into deep veins. The superficial cerebral veins are interlinked with anastomotic veins of Trolard and Labbé. Thus, the superolateral surface of the hemisphere drains into the superior sagittal sinus while the posteroinferior aspect drains into the transverse sinus. The veins of the posterior fossa are variable in course, and angiographic diagnosis of their occlusion is difficult. The entire deep venous system is drained by internal cerebral and basal veins, which join to form the great vein of Galen that drains into the straight sinus. Though variation in the superficial cerebral venous system is a rule, anatomic configuration of the deep venous system can be used as anatomic landmarks. Since thrombosis or surgical sacrifice of the cerebral veins may lead to venous infarction with serious complications, angiographic and surgical anatomy of the venous system should be seriously investigated for each individual patient.

Copyright © 2008 S. Karger AG, Basel

Cerebral Venous System

Understanding cerebral venous system is important to describe the pathophysiology and treatment of cerebral venous thrombosis. Especially when surgery is planned, one has to be able to recognize the major veins and sinuses and to describe their direction of flow. A surgery that involves sacrificing some major cortical veins or subdural bridging veins carries a risk of venous infarction, and vein damage must therefore be kept to a minimum during surgery [1]. The veins of the brain have no muscular tissue in their very thin walls. They possess no valves and emerge from the brain and lie in the subarachnoid space. They pierce the arachnoid mater and the meningeal layer of the dura and drain into the cranial venous sinuses. Most of the cerebral venous drainage collects ultimately into the transverse and sigmoid sinuses of the skull base. The cerebral veins are divided into the superficial and deep groups. The superficial group drains the cortical surfaces. The deep group drains the deep white and gray matter and collects into channels that course through the walls of the ventricles and basal cisterns to drain into the internal cerebral, basal, and great veins [2, 3]. Cerebral venous system can be described in 5 parts: (1) superficial supratentorial cortical veins; (2) dural sinuses and veins; (3) meningeal veins; (4) deep veins; (5) posterior fossa veins.

Superficial Supratentorial Cortical Veins

The superficial veins lie on the surface of the cerebral cortex. They drain mainly into the basal vein of Rosenthal and are considered part of the deep drainage system. Superficial veins drain mainly into four major veins or groups of bridging veins [3, 4]: (1) superior sagittal sinus that receives the superior sagittal group; (2) sphenoparietal sinus and cavernous sinus that receive the sphenoidal group; (3) inferior sagittal sinus and vein of Galen that receive the falcine group, and (4) tributaries of the sinuses related to tentorium cerebelli that receive the tentorial group.

Anatomy

Superior Sagittal Group

This venous sinus lies in the median plane, along the attached border of the falx cerebri. It includes the veins from the superior part of the medial and lateral surfaces of the frontal, parietal and occipital lobes, and from the anterior part of the orbital surface of the frontal lobe.

Sphenoidal Group

These veins drain into the sphenoparietal or cavernous sinus and, less commonly, into the sphenobasal or sphenopetrosal sinuses [5].

Falcine Group

The falcine group is formed by the veins that empty into the inferior sagittal or straight sinus, either directly or through the internal cerebral, basal and great veins. This group is responsible for drainage of the limbic system. The veins on the paraterminal and paraolfactory gyri drain posteriorly toward the anterior cerebral vein.

The anterior parts of the cingulated gyrus and corpus callosum are drained by the anterior pericallosal veins. The posterior part of the cingulate gyrus is drained by the posterior pericallosal vein; the medial part of the parahippocampal gyrus and uncus are drained by the uncal, anterior hippocampal, and medial temporal veins [2, 5].

Tentorial Group

The tentorial group of bridging veins drains into the tentorial sinuses, or into the transverse and superior petrosal sinuses in the tentorial margins [5].

This group includes the temporobasal and occipitobasal veins, and the descending veins, including the vein of Labbé. The vein of Labbé usually enters the transverse sinus.

Normal Angiographic Anatomy

Lateral View

On lateral angiography, 8–12 superior cortical veins can be identified. In the anterior frontal region, cortical veins enter the supra sagittal sinus. Superficial middle cerebral veins can be identified on lateral projections during the venous phase of carotid angiography [6].

The vein of Trolard is also best identified on the lateral view during the mid- to late venous phase of cerebral angiograms. It is a large anatomic cortical vein that courses from the superficial middle cerebral vein to superior sagittal sinus and is the prominent superficial vein on the nondominant side at the late venous phase [6] (fig. 1).

Anterior-Posterior View

On anterior-posterior (AP) projections, the vein of Trolard appears to parallel the inner table of the skull as it curves upward and courses over the cerebral convexity [7].

The vein of Labbé is a large cortical vein that courses from the superficial middle cerebral vein to the transverse sinus and is the prominent superficial vein on the dominant side [7].

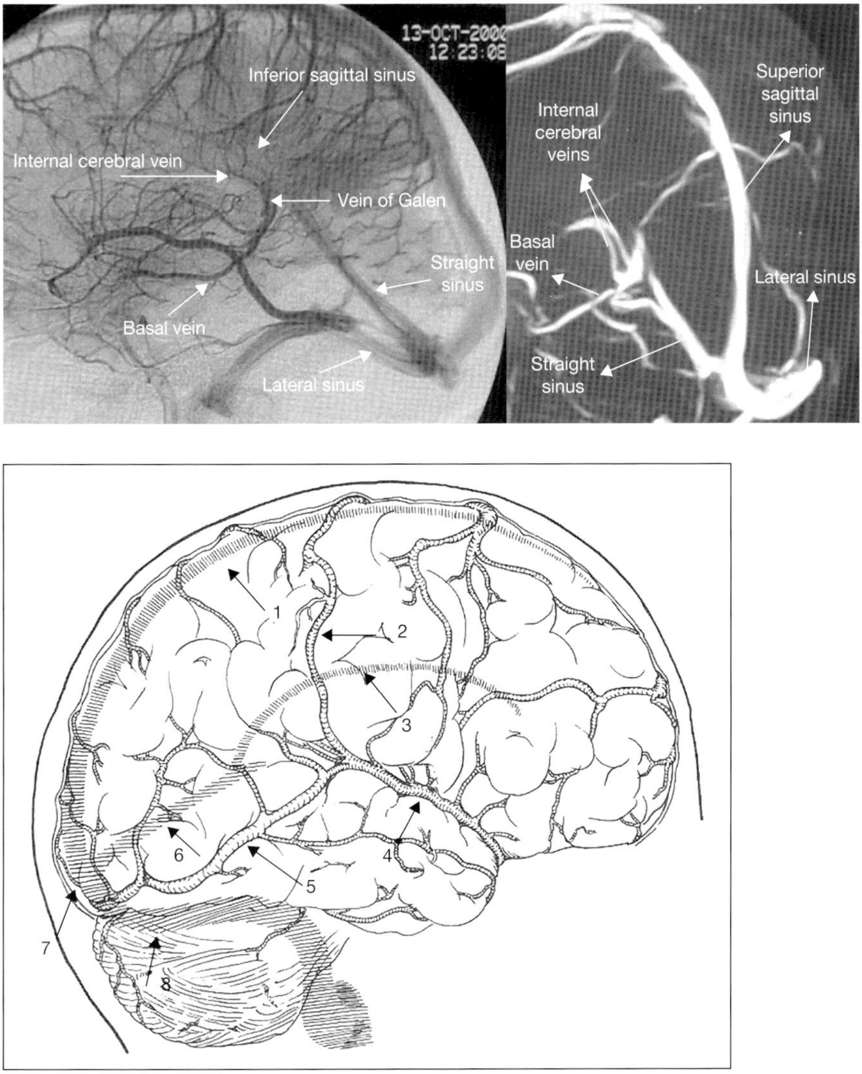

Fig. 1. a Angiographic venous phase of carotid angiogram and MR venography. ***b*** Schematic presentation of the cerebral venous system: superior sagittal sinus (1), vein of Trolard (2), inferior sagittal sinus (3), superficial middle cerebral vein (4), vein of Labbé (5), straight sinus (sinus rectus) (6), torcula herophili (7), transverse sinus (8).

Dural Sinuses and Veins

The dural sinuses receive cerebral veins from the superficial and deep parts. These are: (1) superior and inferior sagittal; (2) straight; (3) transverse; (4) tentorial; (5) cavernous; (6) superior petrosal.

Superior and Inferior Sagittal Sinuses

Superior sagittal sinus superiorly attached to the falx cerebri ends with crista galli. In about 60% of cases, superior sagittal sinus ends by becoming the right transverse sinus. At the termination of the superior sagittal sinus is a dilatation, known as confluence of the sinuses [3]. It is also known as torcula herophili. The superior sagittal sinus also communicates with veins in the scalp through emissary veins that pass through the parietal foramina. The cortical veins may pass directly to the superior sagittal sinus, or they may join the meningeal sinuses, which empty into the superior sagittal sinus.

Inferior sagittal sinus occupies the posterior two thirds of the free inferior edge of the falx cerebri. It ends by joining the great cerebral vein to form straight sinus [3]. The largest tributaries of the inferior sagittal sinus are the anterior pericallosal veins.

Straight Sinuses

This venous sinus is formed by the union of the inferior sagittal sinus with the great cerebral vein. It is attached to the tentorium cerebelli. It may drain into either the transverse sinus or, most commonly, the left transverse sinus.

Transverse Sinuses

These venous sinuses pass laterally from the confluence of the sinuses in the attached border of the tentorium cerebelli. The right transverse sinus, which is usually larger, receives the majority of the drainage from the superior sagittal sinus. So we can guess that the right transverse sinus, right sigmoid sinus and right jugular vein contain blood from the superficial parts of the brain, and the left transverse sinus, left sigmoid sinus and left internal jugular vein contain blood mainly from the deep parts of the brain drained by the internal cerebral, basal and great veins.

Tentorial Sinuses

These sinuses divide into the medial and lateral groups [8]. The medial group drains into transverse sinuses and the lateral group drains into both straight and transverse sinuses.

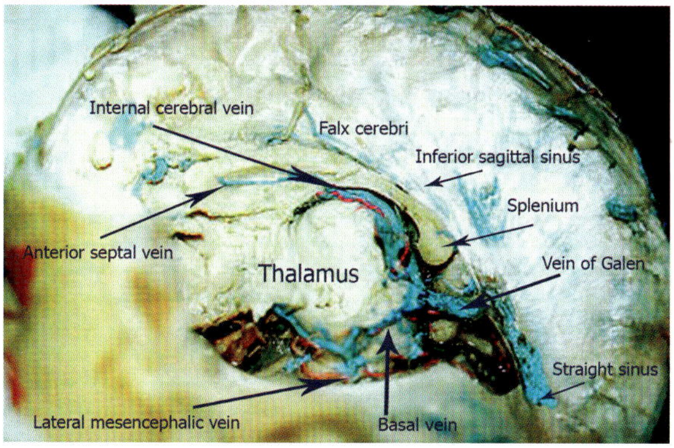

Fig. 2. Cadaveric dissection of deep veins and their drainage at midplane.

Cavernous Sinuses

These large sinuses are about 2 cm long and 1 cm wide. They are located on each side of sella turcica and the body of the sphenoid bone [3]. There are many trabeculae that contain blood channels. Each cavernous sinus receives blood from the superior and inferior ophthalmic veins, the superficial middle cerebral vein in the lateral fissure of the cerebral hemispheres [8]. The cavernous sinus communicates through the superior petrosal sinus with the junction of the transverse and sigmoid sinuses and through the inferior petrosal sinus with the sigmoid sinus.

Superior Petrosal Sinuses

These venous sinuses are small channels that drain the cavernous sinuses. They run from the posterior ends of the cavernous sinuses to the transverse sinuses. Both of petrosal sinuses lie in the attached margins of the tentorium cerebelli. The superficial sylvian veins may empty into an infrequent tributary of the superior petrosal sinus called the sphenopetrosal sinus.

Veins of the lateral hemispheric convexities drain into three major routes: (1) sphenoparietal sinus (sylvian vein); (2) superior sagittal sinus (most prominent Trolard); (3) inferiorly these veins drain into the transverse sinus, and the largest one is called the Labbé vein (fig. 2).

Meningeal Veins

The small venous channels that drain the dura mater covering the cerebrum are called the meningeal veins. They are small sinuses that usually accompany the meningeal arteries. The meningeal veins that accompany the meningeal arteries course between the arteries and the overlying bone. The fact that the artery presses into the veins gives them the appearance of parallel channels on each side of their respective arteries. The largest meningeal veins accompany the middle meningeal artery. The meningeal veins drain into the large dural sinuses along the cranial base at their lower margin and into the venous lacunae and superior sagittal sinus at their upper margin.

Deep Supratentorial Veins

Deep veins are concerned with the drainage of the central structures of the hemispheres, basal ganglia, corpus callosum, pineal region limbic system and thalamus. During operations on the lateral ventricles, the deep veins more commonly provide orienting landmarks than the arteries. The deep veins are divided into a ventricular group, composed of the veins draining the walls of the lateral ventricles, and a cisternal group, which includes the veins draining the walls of the basal cisterns. The deep venous system consists of internal cerebral vein, the basal vein of Rosenthal and their tributaries [9].

Ventricular Group

This group can be divided into two subgroups: (1) Lateral atrial contributions form the common atrial vein that connects to the internal cerebral vein or the vein of Galen. The lateral group deep veins drain caudate nucleus and thalamus and are called the anterior caudate and thalamostriate veins [2]. (2) The medial ventricular group veins drain to the basal vein of Rosenthal. The medial group passes through the outer or forniceal circumference of the fissure.

The medial vein of the frontal horn is represented by the anterior septal veins. The anterior septal vein drains the deep structures of the frontal lobe. It gathers three or five medullary tributaries. It forms the venous angle with the thalamostriate vein. The lateral veins of the frontal horn are anterior caudate veins [2].

The medial veins of the lateral body ventricle are posterior septal veins and the lateral group consists of the thalamostriate, thalamocaudate, and posterior caudate veins. The thalamostriate vein drains the posterior frontal and anterior parietal lobes, caudate nucleus and the internal capsule. The thalamostriate vein is the best known of the subependymal veins because it is the one most frequently seen on angiography. The angle formed by the junction of the thalamostriate and internal cerebral veins at the thalamic tubercle, the venous angle, as seen on the lateral view of the cerebral angiogram, approximates the site of the foramen of Monro [2].

The medial veins of the occipital horn are medial atrial veins and the lateral veins of this group are lateral atrial veins [2].

Cisternal Group

The cisternal group of deep veins drains the area beginning interiorly in front of the third ventricle and extending laterally into the sylvian fissure and backward to include the walls of the chiasmatic, interpeduncular, crural, ambient, and quadrigeminal cisterns.

The area drained by the cisternal group of veins is divided into three regions depending on their relationship to the brainstem and tentorial incisura: an anterior incisural region located in front of the brainstem, a middle incisural region situated lateral to the brainstem, and a posterior incisural space located behind the brainstem.

The major veins of the cisternal group are basal veins and great veins. Basal veins drain anterior, medial and posterior incisural spaces [10].

There are some veins that also drain the deep parts of the brain: (a) Choroidal veins. They drain the deep venous system and go medial to the thalamostriate vein lateral to the fornix and drain into the thalamostriate vein. (b) Thalamic veins. They divide into superior, anterior and inferior thalamic veins. Superior veins drain into the vein of Galen, anterior veins drain into the thalamostriate vein, inferior thalamic veins drain into the interfamilial portion of the thalamus (fig. 3). (c) Internal cerebral veins. The paired internal cerebral veins run from anterior to posterior in the roof of the third ventricle enclosed between two layers of the tela choroidea. This potential space between the two layers is called the cistern of the velum interposition. They drain into the great cerebral vein of Galen [11] (fig. 4). (d) Great cerebral vein of Galen. It receives tributaries from the basal vein of Rosenthal, inferior sagittal sinus. It drains into the straight sinus. It is formed by the union of two internal cerebral vein courses beneath the splenium of the corpus callosum to end at the tentorial apex by uniting with the inferior sagittal sinus to form the straight sinus [11, 12].

Normal Angiographic Anatomy

Deep veins are best identified late in the venous phase, when contrast no longer opacifies the overlying cortical veins.

Lateral View

Medullar veins are best identified on lateral venous phase angiograms. The septal vein follows a straight posterior course as seen on the lateral view. The

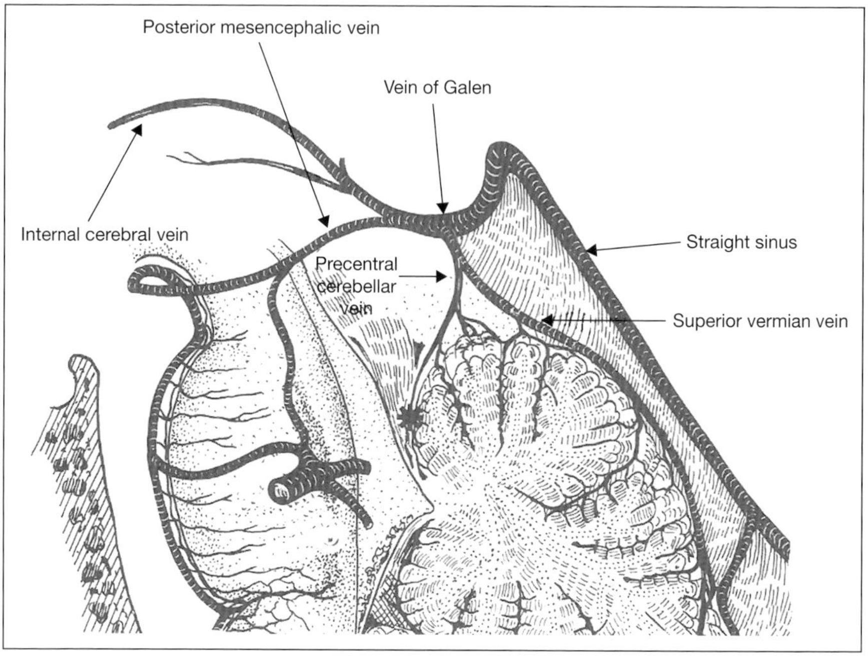

Fig. 3. Posterior fossa veins and their drainage system.

thalamostriate vein receives its caudate and terminal tributaries, and then curves inferiorly to join the septal vein at the foramen of Monroe. The internal cerebral vein extends from the foramen of Monroe posteriorly to the vein of Galen.

The great cerebral vein is also best identified on lateral view. It passes curving posterosuperiorly around the corpus callosum [6].

Anterior View

The thalamostriate vein has a characteristic double curve. The internal cerebral vein is superimposed on the AP view. The basal vein of Rosenthal is characteristic on the AP view. It resembles a frog lying on its back with its legs pointing anterolaterally.

Posterior Fossa Veins

There are three drainage systems that have been described: (a) galenic group; (b) petrosal group; (c) tentorial group.

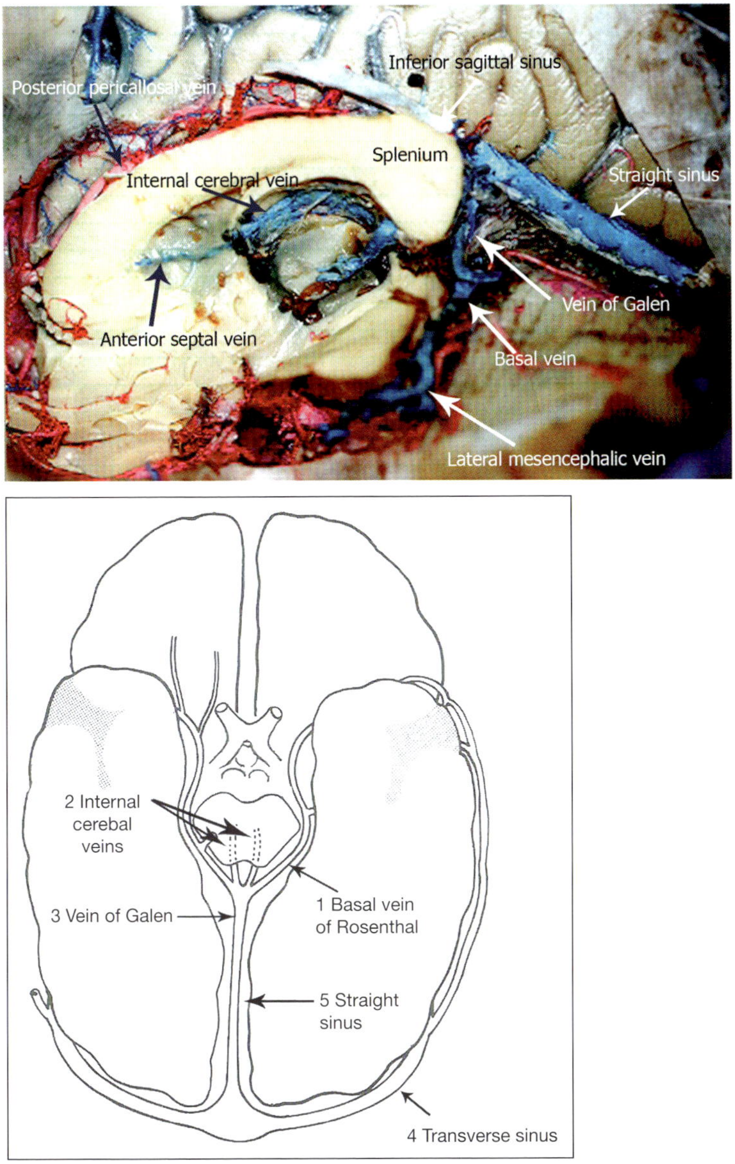

Fig. 4. Cadaveric dissection (***a***), and illustration of the basal vein that drains into the vein of Galen and straight sinus (***b***).

Galenic Group

The galenic group consists of precentral, superior vermian and anterior posterior mesencephalic veins.

The precentral vein is a unique vessel that originates in the fissure between the vermian lingula and central lobule. This vein drains into the vein of Galen after passing the roof of the fourth ventricle.

The superior vermian vein originates near the vermian, curving up and forward along the culmen. The superior vermian vein drains into the vein of Galen [13].

The anterior pontomesencephalic vein consist of many small veins. It passes anterior to the pons and ends with the cerebral peduncle.

Petrosal Group

The most important veins of this group are petrosal veins. They drain into superior petrosal sinus just below the trigeminal nerve.

Tentorial Group

In this group, the important veins are inferior vermian veins. They pass posteriorly along inferior vermis and receive hemispheric veins and usually terminate within tentorial sinuses.

Normal Angiographic Anatomy

Lateral View

The precentral cerebellar vein passes from the roof of the fourth ventricle. The anterior pontomesencephalic vein can be seen behind the clivus; the superior and inferior vermian veins are also seen well on the lateral view [6].

Anteroposterior View

The petrosal vein can be seen well on the AP view. The vermian vein can also be seen. These veins are near the midline [6].

There are some important landmarks in posterior venous system anatomy:

(1) Twining's line: connects the tuberculum sella to the torcular herophili.

(2) Pontomesencephalic vein: anterior border of pons.

(3) Collicocentral point: it helps us find the fourth ventricle. Inflection point where the precentral cerebellar vein changes the upward course slightly posterior.

References

1 Rhoton AL Jr, Yamamoto I, Peace DA: Microsurgery of the third ventricle. 2. Operative approaches. Neurosurgery 1981;8:357–373.

2 Parent A, Carpenter MB: Carpenter's Human Neuroanatomy, ed 9. Baltimore, Williams and Wilkins, 1996, pp 120–128.

3 Moore KL, Dalley AF: Clinically Oriented Anatomy, ed 3. Baltimore, Williams and Wilkins, 1992, pp 637–782.

4 Oka K, Rhoton AL Jr, Barry M, Rodriguez R: Microsurgical anatomy of the superficial veins of the cerebrum. Neurosurgery 1985;17:711–748.

5 Ono M, Ono M, Rhoton AL Jr, Barry M: Microsurgical anatomy of the region of the tentorial incisura. J Neurosurg 1984;60:365–399.

6 Osborn G: Diagnostic Cerebral Angiography, ed 2. Philadelphia, Lippincott Williams & Wilkins, chapter 11, 1999, pp 217–237.

7 Krayenbühl H, Yasargil MG: Cerebral Angiography. London, Butterworth, 1968, p 165.

8 Braun JP, Tournade A, Panisset JL, Straub P: Anatomical and neuroradiological study of the veins of the tentorium and the floor of the middle cranial fossa, and their drainage to dural sinuses. J Neuroradiol 1978;5:113–132.

9 Ono M, Rhoton AL Jr, Peace D, Rodriguez RJ: Microsurgical anatomy of the deep venous system of the brain. Neurosurgery 1984;15:621–657.

10 Huang YB, Wolf BS: The basal vein and its tributaries; in Newton TH, Potts DG (eds): Radiology of the Skull and Brain. St. Louis, CV Mosby, vol 2, 1974, pp 2111–2154.

11 Kılıc T: Angiographic anatomy; in Book of European Association of Neurosurgical Society. New York, Churchill Livingstone, chapter 16, 2002, pp 63–69.

12 Kılıc T, Ozduman K, Cavdar S, Ozek M, Pamir MN: The galenic venous system: surgical anatomy and its angiographic and magnetic resonance venographic correlations. Eur J Radiol 2005;56: 212–219.

13 Yamamoto I, Kageyama N: Microsurgical anatomy of the pineal region. J Neurosurg 1980;53: 205–221.

Türker Kılıç, MD, PhD
Marmara University and Laboratory of Molecular Neurosurgery
Department of Neurosurgery, Institute of Neurological Sciences
Tophanelioglu Street 13/15
TR–34662 Altunizade/Istanbul (Turkey)
Tel. +90 216 327 5249, Fax +90 216 421 4387, E-Mail turkilic@tnn.net

Caso V, Agnelli G, Paciaroni M (eds): Handbook on Cerebral Venous Thrombosis.
Front Neurol Neurosci. Basel, Karger, 2008, vol 23, pp 16–22

Epidemiology of Cerebral Vein and Sinus Thrombosis

Giancarlo Agnelli, Melina Verso

Stroke Unit and Division of Cardiovascular Medicine, Department of Internal Medicine, University of Perugia, Santa Maria della Misericordia Hospital, Sant' Andrea delle Fratte, Perugia, Italy

Abstract

Cerebral venous thrombosis is a serious but potentially treatable cerebrovascular disorder that, unlike arterial cerebrovascular disorder, often affects young adults and children. Cerebral venous thrombosis is a challenging condition for the clinicians because of the wide spectrum of its clinical presentation. Although recognized for more than 100 years, its incidence has been underestimated in the past due to the lack of accurate diagnostic techniques.

Copyright © 2008 S. Karger AG, Basel

Incidence of Cerebral Vein Thrombosis

Cerebral vein thrombosis was first reported more than 100 years ago [1]. Cerebral venous thrombosis affects more commonly the superior sagittal sinus, the lateral sinuses and the transversus sinuses. In about two thirds of the cases the thrombotic process involves more than one cerebral vein. The involvement of cortical veins (Rolandic, parieto-occipital and posterotemporal) is reported in about 40% of the cases of superior sagittal sinus thrombosis. The clinical consequences of the extension of sagittal sinus thrombosis to the cortical veins are variable; generally, this extension is associated with a worsening of the localized edema and with an increased risk of venous parenchymal infarction.

The incidence of cerebral venous thrombosis is only partially known, because of the absence of epidemiologic studies that specifically and systematically addressed this issue. The first data on the incidence of cerebral venous sinus thrombosis were achieved from autopsy series. In the 1960s, Ehlers and colleagues reported 16 cases of cerebral venous thrombosis in about 12,500 autopsies. These autopsy-derived figures caused for years an underestimation of the incidence of cerebral venous thrombosis. Indeed, more recent clinical series reported an estimated incidence about 10 times higher than that found from autopsy series.

Cerebral vein thrombosis can affect adults as well as children and neonates. It is conceivable to report separately on the epidemiology of this disease in adult and pediatric patients. The estimated annual incidence of cerebral venous thrombosis is 3–4 cases per million in adults and 7 cases per million in children or neonates [2, 3]. Among pediatric patients, neonates are the most commonly affected age group. Cerebral venous thrombosis is frequently reported in preschool children. There are no reliable data concerning geographical or racial differences in the incidence of cerebral venous thrombosis. Until the mid-60s, men and women were reported to be equally affected [4]. More recently, cerebral vein thrombosis has been reported to be more common in women, particularly in the age group between 20 to 35 years. This predominance is not evident among children or elderly patients. The female prevalence is probably due to specific age-related conditions such as pregnancy, puerperium and use of oral contraceptives. Data from a study performed in the United States in 1993–1994 estimated that cerebral thrombosis might complicate 11.6 in every 100,000 deliveries.

Etiology

Several inherited and acquired predisposing factors to cerebral venous thrombosis are recognized. However, the cause of cerebral venous thrombosis remains undefined in about one third of the cases. In a series of patients with objectively diagnosed cerebral venous thrombosis, no underlying cause could be identified in 20–35% of patients, even after extensive investigation [5–7].

An initial distinction should be made between infective and noninfective causes. Among the infective causes, infections of the orbit, mastoid, middle ear or face and meningitides are the conditions most commonly associated with cerebral venous thrombosis. Infections of the mastoid or face, in particular, are predisposing factors for a venous thrombosis in the lateral sinuses (transverse or sigmoid). *Staphylococcus aureus*, Gram-negative bacilli and fungi, such as aspergillus, are the most commonly isolated microorganisms in patients with otitis and mastoiditis. Thrombosis of the cavernous sinus is nearly always caused by the infection of paranasal sinuses (ethmoid and sphenoid) or of the orbits. Infective causes probably occur less commonly with modern aggressive antibiotic treatment and nowadays account for no more than 10% of cases [6].

Among the non-infective causes of cerebral venous thrombosis, the most common are cancer, myeloproliferative disorders, dehydration, oral contraceptives, disorders of blood coagulation, collagen diseases and pregnancy or puerperium. In young women, cerebral venous thrombosis occurs more frequently during puerperium than during pregnancy. The mechanical causes such as head trauma, neurosurgical procedures or jugular catheterization are considered to be conditions potentially predisposing to cerebral venous thrombosis. A lumbar puncture can also lead to thrombotic complication of the cerebral veins. A plausible explanation seems to be the reduction in the cerebrospinal fluid pressure due to the procedure where it can generate a dislocation of the brain with traction of its venous structures.

Cerebral venous thrombosis can occur in patients with both inherited and acquired thrombophilic states. Among the inherited conditions, factor V Leiden and prothrombin gene mutations, deficiencies of protein C, S and antithrombin are the most common. It is estimated that these deficiencies account for 10–15% of cases [8, 9]. It has been reported that hyperhomocysteinemia is associated with a 4-fold increased risk of cerebral vein thrombosis [10]. Among the acquired conditions, the antiphospholipid antibodies syndrome is associated with an increased risk of cerebral venous thrombosis [8].

The use of oral contraceptives and, less frequently, hormone replacement therapy has been associated with the increased risk of venous thrombosis, including cerebral venous thrombosis. A recent crossover study reported increases in the levels of factor VII, factor VIII, factor X, fibrinogen and prothrombin fragment 1 + 2 and decreases in the levels of factor V during the use of oral contraceptives. These findings were more pronounced in women on third-generation oral contraceptives (containing desogestrel or gestodene).

The association of acquired predisposing conditions with genetic abnormalities increases the risk of developing cerebral venous thrombosis. Noteworthy, the use of oral contraceptives in carriers of thrombophilic abnormalities appears to be associated with increased risk of cerebral venous thrombosis (OR 22.1; 95% CI 5.9–84.2) [11, 12]. A case-control study compared the prevalence of prothrombotic mutations in 40 women with cerebral venous thrombosis and 120 healthy controls. The study showed that 20% of women with cerebral venous thrombosis had a thrombophilic abnormality (both mutation in the prothrombin and the factor V gene) compared with 7% in the control population. The use of oral contraceptives in women with thrombophilic abnormalities further increases the risk of cerebral venous thrombosis (OR 149; 95% CI 31.0–711.0) [12]. De Bruijn et al. [11] reported a 30-fold increased risk for cerebral venous thrombosis in women with a combination of thrombophilic abnormalities and use of oral contraceptives, as compared to women without either risk factor [11]. A case report described a cerebral venous thrombosis associated with the use of androgens in an otherwise healthy young man [13].

Table 1. Causes of cerebral venous sinus thrombosis

Local
Head injury [18]
Neurosurgery [19]
Meningitides [20]
Arterovenous malformation [21]
Sepsis (sinusitis, mastoiditis, cellulitis) [22, 23]
Stroke and hemorrhage
Space-occupying lesions
Jugular catheterization
Systemic
Dehydration (diabetic ketoacidosis)
Septicemia [24]
Pregnancy and puerperium [5]
Inflammatory bowel disease [25]
Malignancy [26]
Sarcoidosis [27]
Collagen disease (Behcet's syndrome, SLE, Sjögren's syndrome) [28–30]
Homocysteinuria [31]
Nephrotic syndrome [32]
Autoimmune thyroiditis
Drugs
Oral contraceptives [33]
Hormone replacement therapy [34]
Androgens [13]
L-asparaginase [35]
Ecstasy [36]
Blood discrasias
Leukemia [37]
Myeloproliferative disorders
Thrombocythemia
Sickle-cell trait [38]
Paroxysmal nocturnal hemoglobinuria [39]
Thrombotic thrombocytopenic purpura [40]
Heparin-induced thrombocytopenia [40]
Coagulopathies
Protein S, protein C, antithrombin III deficiency [41, 42]
Factor V Leiden [8, 43]
Antiphospholipid antibodies [8]

During pregnancy or puerperium, a significant increase in the risk of cerebral venous thrombosis was associated with caesarian delivery (OR 3.1), increasing maternal age (OR 2.5), presence of comorbidities including hyperhemesis (OR 14.2), intercurrent infections (OR 3.45) and maternal hypertension

(OR 1.9) [14]. A cumulative effect of resistance to activated protein C during pregnancy and decreased protein C levels following caesarian delivery have been recently postulated [15, 16].

Cerebral vein thrombosis, although uncommonly, may be a manifestation of collagen disorders (such as systemic lupus erythematosus, Behcet's disease, Sjögren's syndrome) or inflammatory bowel disease.

Cerebral venous thrombosis can be a complication of nephrotic syndrome and allogeneic bone marrow transplantation [17]. In the case of nephrotic syndrome, renal loss of antithrombin III has been postulated as the potential mechanism for cerebral venous thrombosis.

Hypoxic encephalopathy is a typical cause of cerebral venous thrombosis in the newborns.

The more common causes of cerebral venous thrombosis are listed in table 1.

Conclusion

During the past two decades, the improved awareness of cerebral venous thrombosis and the improvement of neuroimaging techniques have changed consistently the estimation of the incidence of cerebral venous thrombosis. However, despite our improved knowledge, the real incidence of cerebral venous thrombosis remains incompletely defined. The etiology of cerebral venous thrombosis includes several conditions. In about 20–35% of patients with cerebral venous sinus thrombosis, this disease remains idiopathic even after extensive investigation.

References

1 Kalbag R, Woolf A: Cerebral Venous Thrombosis. London, Oxford University Press, 1967.
2 Stam J: Thrombosis of the cerebral veins and sinuses. N Engl J Med 2005;352:1791–1798.
3 de Veber G, Andrew M, Adams C, et al: Cerebral sinovenous thrombosis in children. N Engl J Med 2001;345:417–423.
4 Krayenbuhl HA: Cerebral venous and sinus thrombosis. Clin Neurosurg 1966;14:1–24.
5 Cantu C, Barinagarrementeria F: Cerebral venous thrombosis associated with pregnancy and puerperium. A review of 67 cases. Stroke 1993;24:1880–1884.
6 Ameri A, Bousser MG: Cerebral venous sinus thrombosis. Neurol Clin 1992;10:87–111.
7 Daif A, Awada A, Al-Rajeh S, et al: Cerebral venous thrombosis in adult. A study of 40 cases from Saudi Arabia. Stroke 1995;26:1193.
8 Deschiens M, Canard J, Horellou M, et al: Coagulation studies, factor V Leiden and anticardiolipin antibodies in 40 cases of cerebral venous sinus thrombosis. Stroke 1996;27:1724–1730.
9 Kellett MW, Martin PJ, Enevoldson TP, et al: Cerebral venous sinus thrombosis connected with 20210, a mutation of the prothrombin gene. J Neurol Neurosurg Psychiatry 1998;65:611–612.
10 Martinelli I, Battaglioli T, Pedotti P, et al: Hyperhomocysteinemia in cerebral vein thrombosis. Blood 2003;102:1363–1366.

11 de Bruijn SF, Stam J, Koopman MM, et al: Case-control study of risk of cerebral sinus thrombosis with third generation-oral contraceptives. Cerebral Venous Sinus Thrombosis Study Group. BMJ 1998;316(7131):589–592.
12 Martinelli I, Sacchi E, Landi G, et al: High risk of cerebral vein thrombosis in carrier of a prothrombotic–gene mutation and users of oral contraceptives. NEJM 1998;338:1793–1797.
13 Jaillard AS, Hommel M, Mallaret M: Venous sinus thrombosis associated with androgens in a healty young men. Stroke 1994;25(1):212–213.
14 Laska DJ, Kryscio RJ: Risk factors for peripartum and postpartum stroke and intracranial venous thrombosis. Stroke 2000;31:1274–1282.
15 Cumming AM, tait RC, Fildes S, et al: Development of resistance to activated protein C during pregnancy. Br J Hematol 1995;90:725–727.
16 Griffin JH, Mosher DF, Zimmerman T, et al: Protein C and antithrombotic protein is reduced in hospitalized patients with intravascular coagulation. Blood 1982;60:261–269.
17 Harvey CJ, Peniket AJ, Miszkiel K, et al: MR angiographic diagnosis of cerebral venous sinus thrombosis following allogeneic bone marrow transplantation. Bone Marrow Transplant 2000;25(7):791–795.
18 D'Alise MD, Fichtel F, Horowitz M: Sagittal sinus thrombosis following minor head injury treated with continuous urokinase infusion. Surg Neurol 1998;49:430–435.
19 Ohata K, Haque M, Morino M, et al: Occlusion of the sigmoid sinus after surgery via presigmoidal-transpetrosal approach. J Neurosurg 1998;89:575–584.
20 Jones TH, Bergvall V, Kapelle L: Carotid artery stenose and thrombosis secondary to cavernous sinus thromboses in fusobacterium necrophorum meningitidis. Postgrad Med J 1990;66: 747–750.
21 Pierot L, Chiras J, Duyckaerts C, et al: Intracranial dural arteriovenous fistulas and sinus thrombosis. Report of five cases. J Neuroradiol 1993;20:9–18.
22 Wassermann D: Acute paranasal sinusitis and cavernous sinus thrombosis. Arch Otolaryngol 1967;86:205–209.
23 Grafstein E, Fernandes CM, Samoyloff S: Lateral sinus thrombosis complicating mastoiditis. Ann Emerg Med 1995;25:420–425.
24 Sigsbee B, deck MD, Posner JB: Nonmetastatic superior sagittal sinus thrombosis complicating systemic cancer. Neurology 1979;29:139–146.
25 Musio F, Older SA, Jenkins T, et al: Case report: cerebral venous thrombosis as a manifestation of acute ulcerative colitis. Am J Med Sci 1993;305:28–35.
26 Reddingius RE, Patte C, Couanet D, et al: Dural sinus thrombosis in children with cancer. Med Pediatr Oncol 1997;29:296–302.
27 Byrne JV, Lawton CA: Meningeal sarcoidosis causing intracranial hypertension secondary to dural sinus thrombosis. Br J Radiol 1983;56:755–757.
28 el-Ramahi KM, Al-Kawi MZ: Papilloedema in Behcet's disease: value of MRI in diagnosis of dural sinus thrombosis. J Neurol Neurosurg Psychiatry 1991;54:826–829.
29 Shiozawa Z, Yoshida M, Kobayashi K, et al: Superior sagittal sinus thrombosis and systemic lupus erythematosus. Ann Neurol 1986;20:272.
30 Urban E, Jabbari B, Robles H: Concurrent cerebral venous sinus thrombosis and myeloradiculopathy in Syogren's syndrome. Neurology 1994;44:554–556.
31 Schwab FJ, Peyster RG, Brill CB: CT of cerebral venous sinus thrombosis in a child with homocystinuria. Pediatr Radiol 1987;17:244–245.
32 Akatsu H, Vaysburd M, Fervenza F, et al: Cerebral venous thrombosis in nephrotic syndrome. Clin Nephrol 1997;48:317–320.
33 Buchanan DS, Brazinsky JH: Dural sinus and cerebral venous thrombosis: incidence in young women receiving oral contraceptives. Arch Neurol 1970;22:440–444.
34 Strachan R, Hughes D, Cowie R: Thrombosis of the straight sinus complicating hormone replacement therapy. Br J Neurosurg 1995;9:805–808.
35 Kelly MA, Gorelick PB, Mirza D: The role of drugs in the ethiology of strokes. Clin Neuropharmacol 1992;15:249–275.
36 Rothwell pM, Grant R: Cerebral venous sinus thrombosis induced by 'ecstasy'. J Neurol Neurosurg Psychiatry 1993;56:1035.

37 David RB, Hadfield MG, Vines FS, et al: Dural sinus occlusion in leukemia. Paediatrics 1975;56: 793–796.
38 Feldenzer JA, Bueche MJ, Venes JL, et al: Superior sagittal sinus thrombosis with infarction in sickle cell trait. Stroke 1987;18:656–660.
39 Hauser D, Barzilai N, Zalish M, et al: Bilateral papilloedema with retinal hemorrhages in association with cerebral venous sinus thrombosis and paroxysmal nocturnal hemoglobinuria. Am J Ophthalmol 1996;122:592–593.
40 Meyer-Lindenberg A, Quenzel EM, Bierhoff E, et al: Fatal cerebral venous sinus thrombosis in heparin-induced thrombotic thrombocytopenia. Eur Neurol 1997;37:191–192.
41 Pasquale LR, Moster ML, Schmaier A: Dural sinus thrombosis with abnormalities of protein S and fibrinogen. Arch Ophthalmol 1990;108:644.
42 Roos KL, Pascuzzi RM, Kuharik MA, et al: Post-partum intracranial venous thrombosis associated with dysfunctional protein C and deficiency of protein S. Obstet Gynecol 1990;76:492–494.
43 Bloem BR, van Putten Mj, van der Meer FJ, et al: Superior sagittal sinus thrombosis in a patients heterozygous for the novel 20210A allele of the prothrombin gene. Thromb Haemost 1998;79:235.

Prof. Giancarlo Agnelli
Stroke Unit and Division of Cardiovascular Medicine
Department of Internal Medicine, University of Perugia
Santa Maria della Misericordia Hospital
Via Dottori, Sant' Andrea delle Fratte, IT–06126 Perugia (Italy)
Tel. +39 075 578 6424, Fax +39 075 578 2346, E-Mail agnellig@unipg.it

Caso V, Agnelli G, Paciaroni M (eds): Handbook on Cerebral Venous Thrombosis.
Front Neurol Neurosci. Basel, Karger, 2008, vol 23, pp 23–54

Risk Factors of Cerebral Vein and Sinus Thrombosis

Gabriel R. de Freitas[a], *Julien Bogousslavsky*[b]

[a]Service of Neurology, Universidade Federal Fluminense, Niterói, Brazil;
[b]Department of Neurology, Genolier Swiss Medical Network, Clinique Valmont-Genolier, Glion-sur-Montreux, Switzerland

Abstract

The risk factors for deep venous thrombosis (and for cerebral vein and sinus thrombosis, CVST) differ from those for arterial disease. The risk factors for venous thrombosis are linked to the Virchow triad of stasis of the blood, changes in the vessel wall, and changes in the composition of the blood, especially the first and third of these. Risk factors are usually divided into acquired (e.g. surgery, trauma, pregnancy, puerperium, lupus anticoagulant, malignant disease, and female hormones) and genetic (congenital thrombophilia). However, the separation of genetic and acquired risk factors is somewhat artificial, since they have additive effects and venous thrombosis is often multifactorial. In this review, we discuss acquired risk factors for CVST. These include hormonal changes (e.g. oral contraceptives use, hormone replacement therapy, pregnancy and puerperium), mechanical precipitants (e.g. head trauma, jugular catheterization, surgery, lumbar puncture), local and generalized infections, cancer, acquired prothrombotic states (e.g. hyperhomocysteinemia, nephrotic syndrome), inflammatory diseases (e.g. vaculitis, intestinal inflammatory disease), hematological disorders, neurological diseases (e.g. dural arteriovenous malformations, spontaneous intracranial hypotension), drugs and other situations. However, only some conditions are consistently present in case series, while many appear only in anecdotal reports. Thus, in most situations, a causal link cannot be established. Determining a cause-and-effect relationship is essential for developing preventive, diagnostic, and therapeutic strategies. Therefore, further multicentered, case-controlled studies are crucial for better understanding the pathogenesis of CVST.

Copyright © 2008 S. Karger AG, Basel

Risk factors are characteristics associated with a higher risk of developing a disease. The fact that a characteristic is a risk factor does not necessarily imply that it causes the disease. In some instances, it may be associated indirectly with the disease because it correlates with another variable that determines the disease.

Since diseases often have multiple causes that interact with each other, establishing causality between a risk factor and a disease can be a challenging issue in clinical epidemiology.

Determining a cause-and-effect relationship is essential for developing preventive, diagnostic, and therapeutic strategies. Large randomized controlled trials are generally considered the gold standard in evaluating causality between a risk factor and a disease and the effect of treating (or removing) the risk factor on the incidence of the clinical condition. The great strength of these studies is that, since patients are randomly assigned to either treatment for the putative causal or some alternative treatment (another agent or no exposure at all), the study groups are similar not only in terms of already know determinants of outcome, but also in terms of currently unknown determinants [1]. However, in the case of some risk factors (e.g. smoking), it would not be ethical to randomly assign patients to exposure or nonexposure. In some situations, therefore, a cohort study, in which the investigator identifies exposed and nonexposed groups of patients and follows them to monitor outcome, may provide the best level of evidence, particularly when the information comes from a large database and statistical techniques are used to allow for imbalances due to confounding variables. Nevertheless, an important imbalance, either not measured or unknown to the investigators, may influence the outcome. When the outcome of interest is very rare or takes a long time to develop, case control studies may be used (in fact, these studies are the most commonly used in the setting of cerebral venous and sinus thrombosis, CVST). In these studies, patients who have developed the outcome of interest (cases) are compared with persons who do not have this outcome (controls), but who are otherwise similar to the cases with respect to important determinants of outcome, such as age and sex. Limitations of case-control studies are that a condition may change after the outcome (e.g. see section on hyperhomocysteinemia), a recall bias may influence the results, and, as in cohort studies, unmeasured confounding variables may be responsible for differences. Meta-analysis can provide an objective summary of all the available evidence, but whether this approach is better than large randomized trials is a matter of contention [2].

Risk Factor Classification

The risk factors for venous thrombosis differ from those for arterial disease (table 1). Classical risk factors for arterial disease include hypertension, diabetes, hypercholesterolemia, cigarette smoking, physical activity, alcohol consumption, and diet [3]. The risk factors for venous thrombosis are linked to the Virchow triad of stasis of the blood, changes in the vessel wall, and changes

Table 1. Risk factors for arterial disease, DVT, and CVST

Risk factor	Arterial disease	DVT	CVST
Nonmodifiable			
Age	++	++	––
Gender	+	+	+
Race	++	+	U
Heredity	++	++	++
Modifiable			
Hypertension	++	––	––
Diabetes	++	––	––
Hypercholesterolemia	++	––	––
Obesity	++	+	––
Postmenopausal replacement therapy	+	++	––
Oral contraceptives	+	++	++
Physical activity	++	––	––
Alcohol consumption	++	––	––
Diet	++	––	––
Homocysteine	D	D	D
Immobility	––	++	––
Cancer	––	++	++
Infection	––	++	++

U = Unknown; D = disputable.

in the composition of the blood, especially the first and third of these [4]. Nowadays, risk factors are usually divided into acquired and genetic. Acquired risk factors include obesity, immobilization (including immobilization in plaster casts), surgery, trauma, pregnancy, puerperium, lupus anticoagulant, malignant disease, and female hormones. Genetically determined prothrombotic disorders (congenital thrombophilia) are responsible for a large proportion of cases of venous thrombosis and are discussed in the next chapter. However, the separation of genetic and acquired risk factors is somewhat artificial, since they have additive effects and venous thrombosis is often multifactorial. Thus, even when acquired risk factors are present, congenital thrombophilia should considered. Risk factors can also be divided into modifiable and nonmodifiable.

Risk factors for CVST are, in general, similar to those for deep venous thrombosis (DVT) (table 1), but may not include older age, obesity, hospitalization, and immobility [5].

Hormones

Oral Contraceptives

Several case-control studies [6–14] and one meta-analysis [15] have reported a strong association between oral contraceptives (OCs) and CVST. This association may be responsible for the dramatic shift in the epidemiology of the disease in the last few decades, with CVST changing from a disease affecting men and women equally until the mid 1970s [16] to one predominantly affecting women of childbearing age [17].

In one of the first case-control studies, de Bruijn et al. [7] found that 85% (34 of 40) of women with CVST used OCs versus 45% (1,007 of 2,248) of the control women (odds ratio 13, 95% confidence interval 5–37). Moreover, they found an interaction between OCs and congenital thrombophilia: using estimated population percentages, the odds ratio for women with both risk factors versus women with neither is 34. In another case-control study, Martinelli et al. [8] found an odds ratio of 149.3 (95% confidence interval 31.0–711.0) for women who were taking OCs and who also had the prothrombin gene mutation. In a recent meta-analysis including eight case-control studies of OCs and CVST (263 patients and 2,862 controls), the odds ratio for developing CVST was 5.59 (95% confidence interval 3.95–7.91; $p < 0.001$) in women using OCs [15].

The risk of CVST might vary according to OC formulation, but few studies have addressed this issue. Third-generation OCs seem to carry a higher risk than other OCs [18] and contraceptive patches may confer a risk similar to OCs [19]. Limited data suggest that there is no increased risk of deep vein thrombosis in women who use oral [20] or injectable [21] progestogen-only methods.

Postcoital contraceptive pills, commonly known as the 'morning after pill', are used for emergency contraception and contain substantially higher doses of both estrogen and progestin than standard OCs. However, it is disputable whether emergency contraception may cause venous thrombosis. There exists a single report of CVST after repeated use of postcoital contraceptive pills [22].

The precise mechanism by which OCs increase the risk of CVST is unknown. OC use influences various factors involved in hemostasis. Levels of prothrombin, factors VII, VIII, and X, fibrinogen, and prothrombin fragment 1 + 2 increase and levels of factor V decrease during OC use [23]. OCs can induce activated protein C resistance comparable to the resistance caused by factor V Leiden mutation [24].

Women who suffer from CVST while taking OCs should be counseled about alternative methods of contraception. Some authors suggest that, after 6 months of anticoagulation, these women may be considered for chronic treatment with antiplatelet agents [25].

Hormone Replacement Therapy

There is a huge amount of evidence linking hormone replacement therapy (HRT) with DVT, but there are no significant data (apart from a few anecdotal reports [26, 27]) regarding the relationship between HRT and CVST.

HRT ameliorates symptoms of the menopause and reduces the progression of osteoporosis. Early HRT consisted of an estrogen only, but, due to the strong evidence that unopposed estrogen therapy increased the risk of endometrial cancer, nowadays a progestogen compound, e.g. medroxyprogesterone acetate, is added [28]. Several case-control studies [29–32], cohort studies [33], and randomized controlled trials [34–39], have confirmed the increased risk of DVT in women receiving HRT. A recent meta-analysis of randomized controlled trials found a 2-fold higher risk of venous thromboembolic events (relative risk 2.15, 95% confidence interval 1.61–2.86) in those women randomized to HRT compared with placebo [40]. The high risk of venous thrombosis during the early phases of use suggests that, as with OCs, there is a subgroup of women with a genetic predisposition to thrombosis who are at particular risk when given HRT. Both genetic (factor V Leiden, causing resistance to activated protein C) and acquired (anticardiolipin antibodies) predispositions have been identified in women who presented venous thrombosis soon after hormone use [36, 41].

In the International Study on Cerebral Vein and Dural Sinus Thrombosis (ISCVT), 4.3% of the patients were receiving HRT [42], but it is not known if this is higher than in the general population. It is not clear why hormone replacement is a well-defined risk factor for DVT, but not for CVST. Interestingly, CVST patients are much younger than DVT patients, providing indirect evidence that HRT does not play an important role in CVST.

Pregnancy and Puerperium

Several series of CVST cases occurring during pregnancy and puerperium have been published, most from developing countries [43–50] and Asiatic populations [51, 52]. In one study from Mexico, 60% of the cases of CVST occurred during pregnancy and puerperium [45], whereas, in developed countries, only 5–20% of all cases of CVST are seen in this period. In a study from India, CVST accounted for approximately half of the strokes occurring in young patients and 40% of those occurring in females [47]. A recent study reported a higher incidence of stroke during pregnancy and puerperium in Taiwanese women than in Caucasian populations, CVST being responsible for one quarter of the events [51, 52].

Obstetric CVST is much more common in the puerperium period than in pregnancy, particularly in the first 3 weeks after delivery, with 15% of cases occurring in the first 2 days [45]. When CVST is seen in pregnancy, it can occur in any trimester. It has been suggested that pregnancy/puerperium-related CVST may more commonly have a sudden or acute onset, and a progressive course that tends to become stable in a few days and a better prognosis than nonobstetric CVST [45]. Many risk factors have been implicated in the pathogenesis of peripartum and puerperium CVST. These include dehydration, anemia [45], cesarean delivery, hypertension, infections [48], the mother's age (more common in women aged 15–24 years than in those aged 25–34 years) [49], and thrombophilia [53]. In fact, in a recent study, genetic or acquired thrombophilia was the main cause in 64% (7 of 11) of CVST patients, including protein S deficiency in 4 patients and protein C deficiency and idiopathic thrombocytopenic purpura associated with systemic lupus erythromatosus, and antiphospholipid syndrome in one patient each. Some studies imply that anesthesia (dural puncture) performed for cesarean delivery may be responsible for some cases [54–56].

Mechanical Precipitants (Trauma, Jugular Catheter, Surgery, Lumbar Puncture)

Diverse forms of injury to the central nervous system, i.e. penetrating or close head injury [57–74], neurosurgery [75, 76], electrical injury [77, 78], and lumbar puncture [79–85], have been linked to a higher risk of CVST.

It is not difficult to conceive that CVST may occur after penetrating head trauma in the presence of skull fractures that cross the sinus. In fact, CVST has a reported incidence of 4% after a penetrating head trauma [63]. In addition, there are a number of case reports and several small series of CVST cases associated with skull fractures after closed head injury [60, 62, 67]. In one study, CVST was found in 6.1% (8 of 131) of children with minor or severe head injury (5 children with mild and 3 with severe cranial trauma) [69]. In most cases, the transverse and sigmoid sinuses are involved. Thrombosis can occur in association with mild head injuries in the absence of fractures [54, 68, 74]. The exact mechanism is unknown, but may include compression of the sinuses due to intracranial edema or bleeding, intramural hemorrhages caused by rupture of small sinusoids, injury to the endothelial lining, changes in various components of the blood after head injury, and extension of the thrombus from abrasions of the scalp or injured emissary veins [57, 72]. Some of these patients with mild head trauma have genetic or acquired thrombophilia, and the trauma may act as a trigger for thrombosis [61, 67, 68, 72, 73].

There are some reports of CVST after high-voltage electric injury [77, 78]. The authors postulated that venous thrombosis could be explained by vasospasm and intimal damage provoked by the electric discharge [77]. An alternative or concomitant mechanism for the intimal damage may be related to the heating effect of the electricity.

Surgery [75, 76] and procedures (i.e. jugular catheter) [86–89] involving the head or neck are well known causes of CSVT. Direct sinus lesion, dehydration, transient prothrombotic state, air embolism in patients operated on in a sitting position [90, 91], and thrombophilia [92] have been suggested as putative mechanisms. Central venous access devices are known to be thrombogenic. In patients with central catheters and CVST, the clot begins in the subclavian or jugular vein and propagates intracranially [86–89]. CVST may be more common than previously thought in patients undergoing internal jugular vein resection. The procedure can be necessary in cases of radical neck dissection or even in cases involving benign neoplasms, such as glomus tumors. Among 17 patients subjected to resection, thrombosis of the sigmoid sinus was found in 4 and thrombosis of the transverse sinus in 3 [93]. However, there were no complications, such as intracranial hemorrhage or signs of increased intracranial pressure, in any of these patients. In another study, transverse sinus thrombosis was observed in 5 of 107 patients who underwent suboccipital craniotomy or translabyrinthine craniectomy for resection of a tumor [94]. Even surgical procedures not involving the central nervous system, i.e. cardiac surgery [92, 95] and colectomy for ulcerative colitis [95, 96], have also been reported in association with CVST.

Several reports have proposed that dural puncture may lead to CVST [79–85]. Wilder-Smith et al. [85] described 5 cases of CVST after dural puncture. Three of the 4 patients tested had hereditary activated protein C resistance due to the factor V Leiden mutation, suggesting that thrombophilia may play a role in these cases. One patient was taking an OC. The authors proposed two explanations for thrombosis after dural puncture. In one, a downward pulling or stretching or 'rostrocaudal sagging' effect is exerted on the intracranial contents due to the negative spinal-cranial pressure gradient and this could provoke injury of the cranial nerves, vessels, dura, and brain parenchyma, while the other is cerebral venous vasodilatation triggered by the decreased cerebral spinal fluid pressure, with resultant stasis. Vasodilatation is thought to arise because of the abnormal pressure gradient between the cerebral vasculature and cerebral spinal fluid space. As veins are thin walled and, within certain limits, passively adjust to pressures in and around them, it is likely that a negative pressure on the outside of the vein wall will result in dilatation.

Infection

Infection was one of the main causes of CVST in old series [97]. Fortunately, with the advent of antibiotics, it no longer predominates in recent series. In the ISCVT, infection was a potential cause in only 12.1% (77 of 624)

Table 2. Infective agents related to CVST

Bacterial: septicemia [16, 76], endocarditis [76], typhoid [76], tuberculosis [101–104], *Mycoplasma pneumoniae* [105], *Burkholderia pseudomallei* [106], *Fusobacterium necrophorum* [107–109]
Viral: measles [111], hepatitis virus B and C [114–116], varicella-zoster [112, 113], human immunodeficiency virus [117–119], cytomegalovirus [119]
Spirochetal: leptospirosis [120], syphilis [121]
Parasitic: malaria [122, 123], trichinosis [124, 125]
Fungal: mucormycosis [126–128], aspergillosis [129–134], coccidioidomycosis [135]

of patients [42]. However, it is still a noteworthy mechanism in children (see table 4) [see also the chapter by Yager et al., this vol., pp. 122–131].

Otitis and mastoiditis may be complicated by thrombosis of the adjacent sigmoid and transverse sinuses [95, 98]. Organisms causing infection include *Proteus* species, *Escherichia coli*, *Staphylococcus aureus*, and anaerobes. A condition known as 'otitic hydrocephalus' can occur if the contralateral transverse sinus is hypoplastic, resulting in impairment of absorption of the cerebrospinal fluid, with subsequent intracranial hypertension and papilledema.

Cavernous sinuses thrombosis most commonly follows *S. aureus* infection of the middle third of the face [99]. Other antecedent sites of infection include paranasal (usually sphenoid) sinusitis, dental abscess, and, less often, otitis media.

Superior sagittal sinus thrombosis most frequently accompanies bacterial meningitis or air sinus infection [100]. Causative organisms include *Streptococcus pneumoniae*, *S. aureus*, other streptococci, and *Klebsiella* species.

In one review, septic thrombosis most frequently involved the cavernous sinuses (96 cases), followed by the lateral sinus (64 cases) and the superior sagittal sinus (23 cases) [100].

In addition to local infection, systemic infection can be complicated by CVST. Numerous agents have been reported (table 2) and include bacteria (*Mycobacterium tuberculosis* [101–104], *Mycoplasma pneumoniae* [105], *Burkholderia pseudomallei* [106], *Fusobacterium necrophorum* [107–109], and *Salmonella paratyphi* [110]), viruses (measles [111], varicella-zoster virus [112, 113], hepatitis virus B and C [114–116], immunodeficiency virus [117–119], and cytomegalovirus [119]), spirochetae (*Lepstospira interrogans* [120], and *Treponema pallidum* [121]), parasitae (*Plasmodium falciparum* [122, 123], and *Trichinella spiralis* [124, 125]), and fungi (*Rhizopus* species [126–128], *Aspergillus fumigatus* [129–134], and *Coccidioides immitis* [135]).

Cancer

Central nervous system tumors, as well as systemic malignancies and solid tumors outside the central nervous system, can cause CVST. Central nervous system tumors related to CVST include meningioma, glomus tumor, and medulloblastoma [75]. These tumors often directly compress the veins and sinuses of the brain. Systemic malignancies, such as leukemia, or their treatment by drugs (e.g. asparaginase, thalidomide, corticosteroids) or intrathecal therapy (mechanical injury) [136] may predispose to CVST by a related hypercoagulable state. In terms of solid tumors, CVST frequently results from metastatic disease [137, 138]. Carcinomatous infiltration may also predispose to CVST, but is uncommon [138, 139]. Another rare cause is a paraneoplastic syndrome [140–143]. Tumors can also compress the sinuses without provoking thrombosis; this is especially the case for the superior sagittal sinus, also called the syndrome of 'nonthrombotic occlusion of the superior sagittal sinus'. The clinically distinctive feature is the lack of focal signs during the course of chronic intracranial hypertension [144].

Among 7,029 patients seen in neurologic consultation in the Memorial Sloan-Kettering Cancer Center between January 1994 and April 1998, 0.3% (20) were diagnosed with CVST [136]. Nine of the 20 had hematologic malignancies (6 with acute lymphocytic leukemia and one each with acute myelogenous leukemia/leukemia cutis, chronic myelogenous leukemia, and T-cell leukemia) and 11 had solid tumors [4 had genitourinary cancers (2 prostate, 1 renal cell, and 1 nonseminomatous germ cell tumor), 3 breast cancer, 3 gastrointestinal cancer (2 esophageal and 1 rectal), and 1 melanoma]. The median interval from cancer diagnosis to CVST was 4 months for the patients with hematological malignancies and 20 months for those with solid tumors. This was because CVST in patients with solid tumors often results from metastatic disease and is therefore a late complication, whereas, in hematological malignancies, it is frequently a complication of initial treatment (e.g. asparaginase) or a coagulopathy related to the disease itself. The superior sagittal sinus was the most frequently affected sinus. The authors argued that this sinus may be more susceptible to thrombosis due to its length and location. In addition, a lower pressure and slower blood flow would lead to increased stasis of the blood and subsequent thrombosis. The slower blood flow may lead to tissue hypoxia and a decrease in the clearance of clotting factors. In another study (the ISCVT), 7.4% (46 of 624) of patients with CVST had a malignant disease (20 a solid tumor outside the central nervous system, 18 a hematological malignancy, and 14 a central nervous system tumor) [42].

Acquired Prothrombotic States

Hyperhomocysteinemia

As early as 1969, homocysteine, a sulfur-containing amino acid, was postulated to affect atherosclerotic processes [145]. Increased blood concentrations of homocysteine have been suggested to be a modifiable, independent risk factor for coronary artery disease, stroke, and DVT. Indeed, two meta-analyses found an association between plasma homocysteine and DVT [146, 147]. With regard to CVST, four case-control studies including, altogether, 222 patients and 472 controls supported the homocysteine hypothesis [148–151]. A meta-analysis of these studies found an odds ratio of 4.07 (95% confidence intervals 2.54–6.52; $p < 0.001$) for CVST in patients with hyperhomocysteinemia [15].

Homocysteine is thought to promote thrombosis through enhanced platelet activation, increased thrombin generation, and impaired fibrinolysis, and by causing endothelial dysfunction [152].

Nevertheless, several critical questions remain unanswered in the evolving controversial field of homocysteine and vascular disease. Firstly, two recently published randomized clinical trials (the Heart Outcomes Prevention Evaluation 2, HOPE-2 [153], and the Vitamins and Thrombosis, VITRO [154], studies) failed to show that a lowering of homocysteine by B vitamin supplementation reduces the risk of DVT. Secondly, although results from case-control studies (in which blood for homocysteine measurements was collected after the onset of thrombotic events in cases) support an association between homocysteine and venous disease, data from prospective (or nested-case-control) studies (in which blood for homocysteine measurements was collected before the onset of the thrombotic events) tend to indicate a much weaker relation [146]. This suggests that homocysteine may be an acute phase reactant, rather than a risk factor. Further ongoing randomized trials are needed before we can come to a decision on the benefits and risks of B vitamin supplements for primary or secondary prevention of vascular arterial and venous diseases.

Nephrotic Syndrome

Nephrotic syndrome is characteristically defined as heavy proteinuria (>40 mg/m^2 per hour), hypoalbuminemia (<25 g/l), and clinical edema and can complicate any disease that damages the glomerular membrane basement membrane. While most cases in children are attributable to minimal change glomerulopathy and are referred to as idiopathic nephrotic syndrome, in adults there are numerous etiologies, which include diabetes, amyloidosis, drugs (e.g. nonsteroidal anti-inflammatory drugs), infections (human immunodeficiency virus, hepatitis B and C), neoplasia, and systemic autoimmune diseases.

The hypercoagulability state seen in nephrotic syndrome is multifactorial in origin, and is caused, at least in part, by increased urinary loss of antithrombin III, altered levels and/or activity of proteins C and S, hyperfibrinogenemia due to increased hepatic synthesis, impaired fibrinolysis, and increased platelet aggregability.

CVST caused by nephrotic syndrome was first reported in 1980 [155, 156]. CVST due to idiopathic nephrotic syndrome were recently reviewed by Fluss et al. [157]. Assessing 4 of their own cases (from the Canadian Pediatric Ischemic Stroke Registry) and an additional 17 from the literature, the authors found that, while antithrombin levels were decreased relatively frequently, they were normal in almost half of patients, and that other contributing prothrombotic abnormalities were rarely observed. In the majority of cases, CVST presented during the first flare or within 6 months after the onset of the nephrotic syndrome and the prognosis was good in most patients. Nephrotic syndrome causes between 4.7 and 6% of all cases of CVST in childhood [95, 157].

In adults, it is a rarer cause of CVST (only 0.6%, 4 out of 624, of cases of ISCVT) [42]. CVST related to nephrotic syndrome due to factor V Leiden, systemic lupus erythematosus, human immunodeficiency virus-related nephropathy, or systemic amyloidosis has been reported [158–160].

Antiphospholipid Antibodies

This topic is discussed in the next chapter.

Inflammatory Diseases

Vasculitis

Connective tissue diseases related to vasculitis, such as Behçet's disease [161, 162] and systemic lupus erythematosus [163], are well-recognized causes of CVST. Case reports also suggest a relationship with temporal arteritis [164], Wegener's granulomatosis [165, 166], Sjögren's syndrome [167], rheumatoid arthritis [168], and Churg-Strauss syndrome [169].

In one study, among 250 patients with Behçet's disease, 28% (70) had neurologic involvement and, of these, 35% (25) had CVST [161]. Clinical and neuroimaging features of CVST in these patients were similar to those of patients with CVST of other origins. CVST was the initial feature of Behçet's disease in 2 patients, and in 6 patients thrombosis was contemporaneous with a flare of the disease (aphthous ulcers, arthritis, and fever). Although, in the ISCVT, only 1% (6 of 624) of CVST patients had Behçet's disease [42], in high prevalence areas, such as Saudi Arabia, one quarter (10 of 40) of the CVST cases were caused by Behçet's disease [162].

In many patients with systemic lupus erythematosus, lupus anticoagulant plays a crucial role in the development of CVST. In fact, in one series of 6 patients with systemic lupus erythematosus, 3 patients were found to have lupus anticoagulant [163]. However, other factors, such as defective fibrinolysis, altered antithrombin III function, hyperfibrinemia, or coagulation changes observed during pregnancy or nephritis, in particular during nephrotic syndrome, may be important.

Intestinal Inflammatory Disease

Ulcerative colitis and Crohn's disease are idiopathic inflammatory diseases of the gastrointestinal tract. Thromboembolism is a serious complication of these disorders and reports of CVST in patients with ulcerative colitis appeared 40 years ago [170–174]. Abnormalities of the coagulation cascade, such as factor V mutations, proteins C and S deficiency, prothrombin gene mutation, or hyperhomocysteinemia, in combination with corticosteroid administration, could be key features for increasing the risk of thromboembolic complications. Among 7,199 patients with ulcerative colitis or Crohn's disease followed in one institution, 1.3% (92) developed thromboembolic complications [175]. Nine (10%) of these patients presented cerebral vessel involvement. The frequency of cerebral venous thromboembolic complications in ulcerative colitis patients appears to be greater than that in patients with Crohn's disease. CVST may occur even after remission of the disease [176]. In a recent paper, Umit et al. [177] reviewed 20 cases of CVST and idiopathic inflammatory diseases published in the literature.

Sarcoidosis

CVST is a very rare complication of neurosarcoidosis and only a few cases can be found in the literature [178, 179].

Other Systemic Diseases

Thyroid Disease

Squizzato et al. [180] reviewed 13 patients with combined CVST and thyrotoxicosis. Eight patients had thyrotoxicosis secondary to Graves' disease and 1 secondary to subacute De Quervain thyroiditis, and in 4 the etiology was not specified. The authors claimed that it is unlikely that the association between CVST and thyrotoxicosis is due to chance, and, in addition to thyrotoxicosis, additional procoagulant influences are probably required for thrombosis to develop. Hemodynamic factors, dehydration, and stasis of venous blood flow attributable to goiter may also contribute to the multifactorial pathogenesis of CVST.

Diabetes

Three case reports [181–183] and data on CVST in children (see table 4) suggest that diabetes, acute diabetic hyperglycemia, and ketoacidosis might provoke CVST. There is some evidence that patients with diabetes mellitus have abnormally increased red blood cell adhesiveness to endothelium. However, it is still unclear whether this is a chance association or a causal link. Dehydration may be a confounding factor, and one of the patients had severe iron deficiency anemia [181].

Hematological Diseases

Several hematological disorders have been linked to CVST; these are polycythemia [184], paroxysmal nocturnal hemoglobinuria [185], sickle cell disease [186–191], idiopathic hypereosinophilic syndrome [192], hemolytic anemia [75], and thrombocythemia [193, 194].

The association between iron deficiency anemia and CVST was recently revisited. In a case-control study [195], severe anemia was significantly more frequent in CVST patients (14 of 121) than controls (2 of 120; $p = 0.005$). After multivariate analysis, the association persisted, with an odds ratio of 1.10 (95% confidence intervals 1.01–2.22; $p < 0.05$). Severe anemia was associated with thrombocytosis in 13 of the 16 (81%) and was microcytic in 10 of the 16 (63%). There are three proposed hypotheses why iron deficiency anemia causes thrombosis/ischemia. Firstly, thrombocytosis occurs secondary to iron deficiency anemia and may be associated with a hypercoagulable state; secondly, iron deficiency is thought to contribute to a hypercoagulable state by altering flow patterns in vessels because of reduced red cell deformity and increased viscosity; thirdly, hypoxia secondary to iron deficiency anemia can occur in situations of increased metabolic stress, such as dehydration and infection.

Drugs

In addition to OCs, several drugs have been implicated in the genesis of CVST (table 3). However, only a few are consistently present in case series, while most appear in anecdotal reports. Thus, in most situations, a causal relationship cannot be established. Most reported cases are related to medications for cancer (asparaginase [196–202], tamoxifen [203–205], and thalidomide [206–208]), to hormone stimulation (androgen [209–212], danazol [213], isoflavone [215], and drugs for ovary stimulation [216–218]), stimulation of progenitor cells (erythropoietin [219, 220]), or drugs related to homeostasis (heparin [221], heparinoid [222, 223], and epsilon aminocaproic acid [224, 225]).

Table 3. Drugs associated with CVST

OCs [6–15]
Asparaginase [196–202]
Tamoxifen [136, 203–205]
Thalidomide [206–208]
Androgen [209–212]
Danazol (synthetic androgen) [213]
Oxymetholone (synthetic androgen) [214]
Isoflavone [215]
Erythropoietin [219, 220]
Heparin [221]
Pentosan polysulfate [222, 223]
Epsilon aminocaproic acid [224, 225]
Intravenous immunoglobulin [226]
Clomipramine [227]
Lithium [228]
Sildenafil [229]
Ecstasy [230]
Vitamin A [231]
Steroids [232–235]

Corticotherapy may also be a factor in the genesis of CVST. Numerous cases of CVST have been described after corticosteroid use. Most involved high-dose intravenous corticosteroids (e.g. methylprednisolone for multiple sclerosis), but others occurred after intrathecal infiltration or use for the treatment of multiple myeloma, in particular when combined with thalidomide [206–208]. Corticosteroids appear to be a misleading factor when evaluating the relationship between immunological diseases and CVST. For instance, the association between multiple sclerosis and CVST seems to be due to dural puncture and corticosteroid use in these patients, rather than to the disease per se.

Asparaginase is a bacteria-derived enzyme that provides specific therapy for lymphoid malignancies, such as acute lymphoblastic leukemia. Several cases of CVST linked to asparaginase are found in the literature [196–202]. CVST is a unique feature of asparaginase-related thrombosis and is reported to occur in 1–3% of patients [202]. Some authors suggest the use of anticoagulant treatment or antithrombin concentrates for CVST primary prevention.

Tamoxifen, a selective estrogen receptor modulator with estrogen antagonistic effects in the breast, is an effective treatment for breast cancer. One of its known side effects is systemic thromboembolic events. Seven cases of CVST were recently reported with the use of tamoxifen [136, 203–205]. Tamoxifen may cause thrombosis due to a reduction in levels of antithrombin and protein S.

Thalidomide is an adjunctive therapy for different medical conditions, particularly multiple myeloma. A recent review showed that thalidomide, dexamethasone, or the combination significantly increase the risk of DVT in multiple myeloma patients 2.6-, 2.8-, and 8-fold, respectively [206]. Prophylactic anticoagulation reduces this risk. Only a few cases of CVST linked to thalidomide have been reported [207, 208]. Thalidomide induces apoptosis of tumor cells and this has been shown to have thrombogenic potential. Moreover, it can also damage endothelial cells, resulting in an increased adhesion of tumor cells and platelet clumping and can lead to the production of procoagulant factors, influence the interaction of cancerous cells with these factors, and/or activate platelets and vascular endothelium.

Ovarian hyperstimulation syndrome is the most serious complication of ovarian induction and, in severe forms, is characterized by ovarian enlargement, ascites, electrolyte imbalance, hypovolemia, and hemoconcentration. Several cases of internal jugular vein thrombosis without neurological complications have been reported [216]. However, CVST may also occur [217–218].

Children

CVST in children [95, 98, 236–242] and neonates [98, 243–246] has different causes from those in adults. A large difference is seen in the rate of the most common risk factors between childhood series (table 4), probably reflecting selection criteria bias. The frequency of idiopathic CVST is much lower (less than 5%) [98, 240] than in adults (10%) [42] [see the chapter by Yager et al., this vol., pp. 122–131]. As in adults, most children and neonates have a combination of two or more potential risk factors [98, 245].

Although infection is now a less important cause of CVST, it is still related to a substantial proportion of cases in children. In some series, it was found to be linked to 47% [242] to 74% of cases [94], contrasting with the 12% in adults [42]. Local infections, such as otitis media and mastoiditis, are particularly common in preschool children. Dehydration, not necessarily in the presence of infection, seems to be 10 times more common in children (21%) [94, 240] than in adults (1.9%) [42].

Risk factors in neonates are different from those in children. In one large study, perinatal complications were responsible for half of the cases (35 of 69 cases); these included hypoxia at birth (in 30), premature rupture of membranes (in 4), maternal infection (in 4), placental abruption (in 2), and gestational diabetes (in 2) [240]. Dehydration was also an important cause, being implicated in 30% of the cases. Another study pointed out that maternal gestational risk factors may be a significant factor in cases of neonatal CVST, particularly in children who present in the 1st week of life: 26% (10) of 38 women with babies

Table 4. Risk factors of CVST in children in the four largest clinical series

First author	Cases	Infection	Trauma	Chronic disease	Dehydration	Thrombophilia	Drug	None
DeVeber, 2001 [240]	91[1]	25 (27%; 21 head or neck, 4 septicemia)	NR	55 (60%; 21 connective tissue disease, 18 hematologic disorder, 12 cancer, 8 cardiac disease, 5 disorder requiring indwelling catheter)	19 (21%)	29 (39%)	14 (19%; 11 asparaginase, 3 OCs)	3 (3%)
Heller, 2003 [98]	109[2]	44 (29%; 14 mastoiditis, 5 otitis, 6 meningitis, 8 septicemia, 5 sinusitis, 2 varicella zoster infection, 4 infectious gastroenteritis)	10 (7%)	33 (22%; 27 leukemia or lymphoma, 1 colitis ulcerosa, 2 diabetes, 2 obesity, 1 nephrotic syndrome)[3]	NR	84 (56%)	37 (25%; 33 steroids: 27 for leukemia or lymphoma induction therapy, concomitant with asparaginase, 5 for induction of fetal lung maturation in preterm labor, 1 for colitis ulcerosa), 4 OCs	18

Kenet, 2004 [242]	38	18 (47%) (septicemia, varicella, acute encephalitis)[4]	NR	8 (21%; 4 cardiac disease, 2 systemic lupus erythematosus, 1 homocysteinuria, 1 nephrotic syndrome)	NR	16 (42%)	1 (2.6%; OC)	7 (18%)
Sébire, 2005 [95]	42	31 (74%; 20 mastoiditis, 1 sinusitis, 10 other)	2 (4%)	17 (40%; 3 nephrotic syndrome, 2 cardiac disease, 2 systemic lupus erythematosus, 2 sickle cell disease, 2 brain tumors, 2 hydrocephalus with recent shunt surgery, 2 leukemia, 1 inflammatory bowel disease, 1 thalassemia)	9 (21%)	18 (62%) of the 29 screened	NR	0

NR = Not reported.
[1]Sixty-nine neonates not included.
[2]Data from 40 neonates could not be analyzed separately from 109 older children (28 days to 18 years), so the percentages were calculated using the 149 patients.
[3]Calculated by the authors of this chapter.
[4]Numbers not specified.

with CVST had preeclampsia or hypertension and 26% (10) had gestational diabetes or chronic diabetes [246]. Major neonatal medical conditions, including congenital heart disease and disseminated intravascular coagulation, may also play an important role in the etiology of the disease [245].

Neurological Disorders

Various neurological disorders of vascular and nonvascular origin have been linked with CVST. Cerebral vascular diseases include ischemic stroke [75, 76], hemorrhagic stroke [75, 76], arteriovenous malformations [247], and dural arteriovenous malformations [248–268]. Nonvascular diseases comprise neurosurgery, head injury, meningitis, abscess, empyema [74], intracranial tumors, intracranial metastasis, carcinomatous infiltration, glomus tumor [247], porencephaly, arachnoid cysts [247], multiple sclerosis [269–276], and spontaneous intracranial hypotension [277–282]. Most of these have already been discussed above. We will briefly discuss dural arteriovenous fistulas, multiple sclerosis, and spontaneous intracranial hypotension.

Dural Arteriovenous Malformations

Since the 1980s, several case reports and several small series have described an association between dural arteriovenous malformations and CVST [248–268]. In a recent paper, Tsai et al. [268] found that 39% (27 of 69) of patients with dural arteriovenous malformations also had CVST. On analyzing the features of patients with dural arteriovenous malformations with or without CVST, they found no significant differences between the two groups with regard to sex or location or type of malformation.

One hypothesis proposed for the link between the two diseases is based on the physiological arteriovenous shunts between the meningeal arterial networks and the dural venous sinuses. CVST could result in an increase in sinus and venous pressure, opening these channels to create dural arteriovenous fistulas. An alternative hypothesis, supported mainly by animal models, is that venous hypertension induced by a CVST may reduce cerebral perfusion and lead to ischemia, followed by angiogenesis. The aberrant angiogenic activity of the dural blood vessels would then result in arteriovenous shunting.

Multiple Sclerosis

At least 13 patients with both multiple sclerosis and CVST have been reported since 1994 [83, 269–276]. All of these, except 2 reported by Vanderberghe et al. [274], had undergone lumbar puncture and/or received high-dose intravenous methylprednisolone a few days prior to CVST. These authors argued that patients with multiple sclerosis could have a higher risk of CVST since the relationship between plaques and brain parenchyma blood vessels is close, with an inflammatory infiltration around small or medium-sized veins, and that several immunological mechanisms lead to inflammation of the blood vessel wall and to increased permeability of the blood-brain barrier [274]. Nevertheless, a fortuitous association of the two diseases cannot be discounted.

Spontaneous Intracranial Hypotension

Spontaneous intracranial hypotension, i.e. intracranial hypotension occurring in the absence of any recent dural puncture or known tear, is a rare condition. In 2004, Berroir et al. [277] reported 2 cases of spontaneous intracranial hypotension complicated by CVST. The diagnosis was established before lumbar puncture. Potential risk factors for CVST were prolonged bed rest due to orthostatic headache and prothrombotic conditions, such as hereditary thrombophilia in one of the patients, and possibly the association of heavy smoking and oral progestogens in the other. In the same year, Sopelana et al. [278] reported an additional case of a 56-year-old man, a smoker and with hypercholesterolemia, who presented spontaneous intracranial hypotension and transverse, sigmoid jugular and superior longitudinal sinus thrombosis. Complementary studies did not disclose any conventional cause for CVST. The pathogenic connection between the two entities could be similar to that proposed for dural puncture (see above). An alternative supposition is that the velocity of the blood flow in the dural sinuses may be reduced in spontaneous intracranial hypotension because of dilatation of the venous system which compensates the cerebral spinal fluid loss, thus predisposing to thrombosis. A few extra cases were published in recent years [279–282].

Arterial Risk Factors

Red clot (fibrin-rich) and white clot (platelet-rich) classically represent two separate pathophysiological entities, which are, respectively, arterial and venous thromboembolic diseases. With arterial disease, the processes of endothelial damage/dysfunction, inflammation, and thrombogenesis (with coagulation/platelet abnormalities) are well-recognized, resulting in the dynamic, progressive disease of atherothrombotic disease. In reality, thrombogenesis and atherogenesis are closely related. Since atherosclerosis is known to involve platelet and coagulation activation, as well as fibrin turnover, it is not unreasonable to suggest a plausible pathophysiological link between venous thromboembolism and atherosclerosis [283]. Platelet and coagulation activation are inseparable, reciprocally self-amplifying processes. Goon and Lip [283] argued that, instead of a 'cause and effect' scenario, a more likely one assumes that the same 'biological trigger' is responsible for activating the coagulation and inflammatory pathways in both arterial and venous thromboembolism. This would be in line with the elevated levels of inflammatory mediators seen in both conditions, as well as the increased risk of cardiovascular events in patients with idiopathic venous thromboembolism.

Recent studies suggest that the two conditions have many risk factors in common, including older age, obesity, diabetes mellitus, hyperlipidemia, and hypertension [284, 285]. Furthermore, among individuals aged 65 years or older, statin use is associated with a 22% reduction in the risk of DVT [286] and a diet including more vegetables, fruit, and fish and less red and processed meat is associated with a 30–45% lower incidence of the disease [287]. Further data suggesting a link between arterial and venous pathologies come from the Multiple Environmental and Genetic Assessment case-control study including men and women aged 18–70, in which moderate exercise was associated with a lower risk of venous thrombosis of the arm [288]. However, some results of other large cohort studies, such as the Atherosclerosis Risk in Communities study [289] and the Cardiovascular Health Study [290], do not support this view. If the pathogenesis and risk factors of venous thromboembolism are less well understood than those of arterial disease, far less information is available for CVST. The infrequency of the disease and the fact that certain well-established risk factors for venous thromboembolism (e.g. age and obesity) do not play a role in CVST limit our understanding of the disease. Further multicentered, case-controlled studies are crucial for determining the etiology of, and, therefore, methods for the prevention of, CVST.

References

1 Levine M, Walter S, Lee H, Haines T, Holbrook A, Moyer V: Users' guides to the medical literature. IV. How to use an article about harm. Evidence-Based Medicine Working Group. JAMA 1994;271:1615–1619.

2 Baillar JC III: The promise and problems of meta-analysis. N Eng J Med 1997;337:559–561.

3 de Freitas GR, Bogousslavsky J: Primary stroke prevention. Eur J Neurol 2001;8:1–15.

4 Rosendaal FR: Venous thrombosis: a multicausal disease. Lancet 1999;353:1167–1173.

5 Cushman M: Epidemiology and risk factors for venous thrombosis. Semin Hematol 2007;44:62–69.

6 Martinelli I, Landi G, Merati G, Cella R, Tosetto A, Mannucci PM: Factor V gene mutation is a risk factor for cerebral venous thrombosis. Thromb Haemost 1996;75:393–394.

7 de Bruijn SF, Stam J, Koopman MM, Vandenbroucke JP; for the Cerebral Venous Sinus Thrombosis Study Group: Case-control study of risk of cerebral sinus thrombosis in oral contraceptive users and in [correction of who are] carriers of hereditary prothrombotic conditions. BMJ 1998;316:589–592. [Erratum, BMJ 1998;316:822.]

8 Martinelli I, Sacchi E, Landi G, Taioli E, Duca F, Mannucci PM: High risk of cerebral-vein thrombosis in carriers of a prothrombin-gene mutation and in users of oral contraceptives. N Engl J Med 1998;338:1793–1797.

9 Reuner KH, Ruf A, Grau A: Prothrombin gene G20210–A transition is a risk factor for cerebral venous thrombosis. Stroke 1998;29:1765–1769.
10 Martinelli I, Battaglioli T, Pedotti P, Cattaneo M, Mannucci PM: Hyperhomocysteinemia in cerebral vein thrombosis. Blood 2003;102:1363–1366.
11 Gadelha T, Andre C, Juca AA, Nucci M: Prothrombin 20210A and oral contraceptive use as risk factors for cerebral venous thrombosis. Cerebrovasc Dis 2005;19:49–52.
12 Rodrigues CA, Rocha LK, Morelli VM, Franco RF, Lourenco DM: Prothrombin 20210A mutation, and not factor V Leiden mutation, is a risk factor for cerebral venous thrombosis in Brazilian patients. J Thromb Haemost 2004;2:1211–1212.
13 Cantu C, Alonso E, Jara A, Martinez L, Rios C, Fernandez Mde L, Garcia I, Barinagarrementeria F: Hyperhomocysteinemia, low folate and vitamin B12 concentrations, and methylene tetrahydrofolate reductase mutation in cerebral venous thrombosis. Stroke 2004;35:1790–1794.
14 Ventura P, Cobelli M, Marietta M, Panini R, Rosa MC, Salvioli G: Hyperhomocysteinemia and other newly recognized inherited coagulation disorders (factor V Leiden and prothrombin gene mutation) in patients with idiopathic cerebral vein thrombosis. Cerebrovasc Dis 2004;17:153–159.
15 Dentali F, Crowther M, Ageno W: Thrombophilic abnormalities, oral contraceptives, and risk of cerebral vein thrombosis: a meta-analysis. Blood 2006;107:2766–2773.
16 Krayenbühl HA: Cerebral venous and sinus thrombosis. Clin Neurosurg 1966;14:1–24.
17 Stam J: Thrombosis of the cerebral veins and sinuses. N Engl J Med 2005;352:1791–1798.
18 de Bruijn SF, Stam J, Vandenbroucke JP: Increased risk of cerebral venous sinus thrombosis with third-generation oral contraceptives. Lancet 1998;351:1404.
19 Jick SS, Jick H: Cerebral venous sinus thrombosis in users of four hormonal contraceptives: levonorgestrel-containing oral contraceptives, norgestimate-containing oral contraceptives, desogestrel-containing oral contraceptives and the contraceptive patch. Contraception 2006;74: 290– 292.
20 World Health Organization. Collaborative Study of Cardiovascular Disease and Steroid Hormone Contraception. Cardiovascular disease and use of oral and injectable progestogen-only contraceptives and combined injectable contraceptives. Results of an international, multicenter, case-control study. Contraception 1998;57:315–324.
21 International Collaborative Post-marketing Surveillance of Norplant: Postmarketing surveillance of Norplant contraceptive implants. II. Non-reproductive health. Contraception 2001;63: 187–209.
22 Horga A, Santamarina E, Quilez A, de Francisco J, Garcia-Martinez R, Alvarez-Sabin J: Cerebral venous thrombosis associated with repeated use of emergency contraception. Eur J Neurol 2007;14:e5.
23 Middeldorp S, Meijers JC, van den Ende AE, van Enk A, Bouma BN, Tans G, Rosing J, Prins MH, Buller HR: Effects on coagulation of levonorgestrel- and desogestrel-containing low dose oral contraceptives: A cross-over study. Thromb Haemost 2000;84:4–8.
24 Rosing J, Tans G, Nicolaes GA, Thomassen MC, van Oerle R, van der Ploeg PM, Heijnen P, Hamulyak K, Hemker HC: Oral contraceptives and venous thrombosis: different sensitivities to activated protein C in women using second- and third-generation oral contraceptives. Br J Haematol 1997;97:233–238.
25 Saadatnia M, Tajmirriahi M: Hormonal contraceptives as a risk factor for cerebral venous and sinus thrombosis. Acta Neurol Scand 2007;115:295–300.
26 Knox AM, Brophy BP, Sage MR: Cerebral venous thrombosis in association with hormonal supplement therapy. Clin Radiol 1990;41:355–357.
27 Strachan R, Hughes D, Cowie R: Thrombosis of the straight sinus complicating hormone replacement therapy. Br J Neurosurg 1995;9:805–808.
28 Rosendaal FR, Helmerhorst FM, Vandenbroucke JP: Oral contraceptives, hormone replacement therapy and thrombosis. Thromb Haemost 2001;86:112–123.
29 Daly E, Vessey MP, Hawkins MM, Carson JL, Gough P, Marsh S: Risk of venous thromboembolism in users of hormone replacement therapy. Lancet 1996;348:977–980.
30 Jick H, Derby LE, Wald Myers M, Vasilakis C, Newton KM: Risk of hospital admission for idiopathic venous thromboembolism among users of postmenopasusal oestrogens. Lancet 1996;348: 981–983.

31 Varas-Lorenzo C, Garcia-Rodriguez LA, Cattaruzzi C, Troncon MG, Agostinis L, Perez-Gutthann S: Hormone replacement therapy and the risk of hospitalization for venous thromboembolism: a population-based study in southern Europe. Am J Epidemiol 1998;147:387–390.
32 Perez-Gutthann S, Garcia-Rodriguez LA, Castellsague J, Duque-Oliart A: Hormone replacement therapy and risk of venous thromboembolism: population based case-control study. Br Med J 1997;314:796–800.
33 Høibraaten E, Abdelnoor M, Sandset PM: Hormone replacement therapy with estradiol and risk of venous thromboembolism–a population-based case-control study. Thromb Haemost 1999;82: 1218–1221.
34 Grodstein F, Stampfer MJ, Goldhaber SZ, Manson JE, Colditz GA, Speizer FE, Willett WC, Hennekens CH: Prospective study of exogenous hormones and risk of pulmonary embolism in women. Lancet 1996;348:983–987.
35 Hulley S, Grady D, Bush T, Furberg C, Herrington D, Riggs B, Vittinghoff E: Randomized trial of estrogen plus progestin for secondary prevention of coronary heart disease in postmenopausal women. Heart and Estrogen/progestin Replacement Study (HERS) Research Group. JAMA 1998;280:605–613.
36 Høibraaten E, Qvigstad E, Arnesen H, Larsen S, Wickstrøm E, Sandset PM: Increased risk of recurrent venous thromboembolism during hormone replacement therapy – results of the randomized, double-blind, placebo controlled estrogen in venous thromboembolism trial (EVTET). Thromb Haemost 2000;84:961–967.
37 Grady D, Wenger NK, Herrington D, Khan S, Furberg C, Hunninghoke D, Vittinghoff E, Hulley S: Postmenopausal hormone therapy increases risk for venous thromboembolic disease. Ann Intern Med 2000;132:689–696.
38 Rossouw JE, Anderson GL, Prentice RL, LaCroix AZ, Kooperberg C, Stefanick ML, Jackson RD, Beresford SA, Howard BV, Johnson KC, Kotchen JM, Ockene J; for the Writing Group for the Women's Health Initiative Investigators: Risks and benefits of estrogen plus progestin in healthy postmenopausal women: principal results from the Women's Health Initiative randomized controlled trial. JAMA 2002;288:321–333.
39 Cushman M, Kuller LH, Prentice R, Rodabough RJ, Psaty BM, Stafford RS, Sidney S, Rosendaal FR; for the Women's Health Initiative Investigators: Estrogen plus progestin and risk of venous thrombosis. JAMA 2004;292:1573–1580.
40 Gabriel-Sánchez R, Carmona L, Roque M, Sánchez-Gómez LM, Bonfill X: Hormone replacement therapy for preventing cardiovascular disease in post-menopausal women. Cochrane Database of Systematic Reviews 2005, Issue 2. Art. No.: CD002229.
41 Lowe G, Woodward M, Vessey M, Rumley A, Gough P, Daly E: Thrombotic variables and risk of idiopathic venous thromboembolism in women aged 45–64 years: relationships to hormone replacement therapy. Thromb Haemost 2000;83:530–535.
42 Ferro JM, Canhao P, Stam J, Bousser MG, Barinagarrementeria F; ISCVT Investigators: Prognosis of cerebral vein and dural sinus thrombosis: results of the International Study on Cerebral Vein and Dural Sinus Thrombosis (ISCVT). Stroke 2004;35:664–670.
43 Bansal BC, Gupta RR, Prakash C: Stroke during pregnancy and puerperium in young females below the age of 40 years as a result of cerebral venous/venous sinus thrombosis. Jpn Heart J 1980;21:171– 183.
44 Srinivasan K: Cerebral venous and arterial thrombosis in pregnancy and puerperium. A study of 135 patients. Angiology 1983;34:731–746.
45 Cantu C, Barinagarrementeria F: Cerebral venous thrombosis associated with pregnancy and puerperium: review of 67 cases. Stroke 1993;24:1880–1884.
46 Ben Hamouda-M'Rad I, Mrabet A, Ben Hamida M: Thromboses veineuses et infarctus arteriels cerebraux au cours de la grossesse et du post-partum. Une serie de 60 cas. Rev Neurol (Paris) 1995;151:563–568.
47 Panagariya A, Maru A: Cerebral venous thrombosis in pregnancy and puerperium–a prospective study. J Assoc Physicians India 1997;45(11):857–859.
48 Lanska DJ, Kryscio RJ: Stroke and intracranial venous thrombosis during pregnancy and puerperium. Neurology 1998;51:1622–1628.

49 Lanska DJ, Kryscio RJ: Risk factors for peripartum and postpartum stroke and intracranial venous thrombosis. Stroke 2000;31:1274–1282.
50 Francois P, Fabre M, Lioret E, Jan M: Vascular cerebral thrombosis during pregnancy and postpartum. Neurochirurgie 2000;46:105–109.
51 Jeng JS, Tang SC, Yip PK: Incidence and etiologies of stroke during pregnancy and puerperium as evidenced in Taiwanese women. Cerebrovasc Dis 2004;18:290–295.
52 Jeng JS, Tang SC, Yip PK: Stroke in women of reproductive age: comparison between stroke related and unrelated to pregnancy. J Neurol Sci 2004;221:25–29.
53 Carhuapoma JR, Mitsias P, Levine SR: Cerebral venous thrombosis and anticardiolipin antibodies. Stroke 1997;28:2363–2369.
54 Younker D, Jones MM, Adenwala J, Citrin A, Joyce TH 3rd: Maternal cortical vein thrombosis and the obstetric anesthesiologist. Anesth Analg 1986;65:1007–1112.
55 Ravindran RS, Zandstra GC, Viegas OJ: Postpartum headache following regional analgesia: a symptom of cerebral venous thrombosis. Can J Anaesth 1989;36:705–707.
56 Kapessidou Y, Vokaer M, Laureys M, Bier JC, Boogaerts JG: Case report: cerebral vein thrombosis after subarachnoid analgesia for labour. Can J Anaesth 2006;53:1015–1019.
57 Kinal M: Traumatic thrombosis of dural venous sinuses in closed head injuries. J Neurosurg 1967;27:142–145.
58 Bjornebrink J, Liliequist B: Traumatic lateral sinus thrombosis. Report of two cases. Angiology 1976;27:688–697.
59 Ghorayeb B, Yeakley J, Hall J, Jones E: Unusual complications of temporal bone fractures. Arch Otolaryngol Head Neck Surg 1987;113:749–753.
60 Mas JL, Meder JF, Meary E, Bousser MG: Magnetic resonance imaging in lateral sinus hypoplasia and thrombosis. Stroke 1990;21:1350–1356.
61 Rich C, Gill JC, Wernick S, Konkol RJ: An unusual cause of cerebral venous thrombosis in a four-year-old child. Stroke 1993;24:603–605.
62 Taha JM, Crone KR, Berger TS, Becket WW, Prenger EC: Sigmoid sinus thrombosis after closed head injury in children. Neurosurgery 1993;32:541–545.
63 Ochagavia AR, Boque MC, Torre C, Alonso S, Sirvent JJ: Dural venous sinus thrombosis due to cranial trauma. Lancet 1996;347:1564.
64 D'Alise MD, Fichtel F, Horowitz M: Sagittal sinus thrombosis following minor head injury treated with continuous urokinase infusion. Surg Neurol 1998;49:430–435.
65 Ferrera PC, Pauze DR, Chan L: Sagittal sinus thrombosis after closed head injury. Am J Emerg Med 1998;16:382–385.
66 Kuether TA, ONeill O, Nesbit GM, Barnwell SL: Endovascular treatment of traumatic dural sinus thrombosis: case report. Neurosurgery 1998;42:1163–1166.
67 Holzmann D, Huisman TA, Linder TE: Lateral dural sinus thrombosis in childhood. Laryngoscope 1999;109:645–651.
68 Saneto RP, Samples S, Kinkel RP: Traumatic intracerebral venous thrombosis associated with an abnormal golf swing. Headache 2000;40:595–598.
69 Stiefel D, Eich G, Sacher P: Posttraumatic dural sinus thrombosis in children. Eur J Pediatr Surg 2000;10:41–44.
70 Kumar GS, Chacko AG, Chacko M: Superior sagittal sinus and torcula thrombosis in minor head injury. Neurol India 2004;52:123–124.
71 Rottger C, Trittmacher S, Gerriets T, Kaps M, Stolz E: Sinus thrombosis after a jump from a small rock and a sneezing attack: minor endothelial trauma as a precipitating factor for cerebral venous thrombosis? Headache 2004;44:812–825.
72 Muthukumar N: Cerebral venous sinus thrombosis and thrombophilia presenting as pseudotumour syndrome following mild head injury. J Clin Neurosci 2004;11:924–927.
73 Muthukumar N: Uncommon cause of sinus thrombosis following closed mild head injury in a child. Childs Nerv Syst 2005;21:86–88.
74 Yuen HW, Gan BK, Seow WT, Tan HK: Dural sinus thrombosis after minor head injury in a child. Ann Acad Med Singapore 2005;34:639–641.
75 Barnett HJM, Hyland HH: Non-infective intracranial venous thrombosis. Brain 1953;76:36–49.
76 Garcin R, Pestel M: Thrombophlébites cérébrales. Paris, Masson, 1949.

77 Patel A, Lo R: Electric injury with cerebral venous thrombosis. Stroke 1993;24:903–905.
78 Sure U, Kleihues P: Intracerebral venous thrombosis and hematoma secondary to high-voltage brain injury. J Trauma 1997;42:1161–1164.
79 Lega BC, Yoshor D: Postoperative dural sinus thrombosis in a patient in a hypercoagulable state. Case report. J Neurosurg 2006;105:772–774.
80 Schou J, Scherb M: Postoperative sagittal sinus thrombosis after spinal anesthesia. Anesth Analg 1986;65:541–542.
81 Hubbert CH: Dural puncture headache suspected, cortical vein thrombosis diagnosed. Anesth Analg 1987;66:285.
82 Brugeilles H, Peinisson-Besnier I, Pasco I, Ollic P, Lejeune P, Mercier P: Cerebral venous thrombosis after myelography with iopamidol. Neuroradiology 1996;38:534–536.
83 Borum SE, Naul LG, McLeskey CH: Postpartum dural venous sinus thrombosis after postdural puncture headache and epidural blood patch. Anesthesiology 1997;86:487–490.
84 Aidi S, Chaunu MP, Biousse V, Bousser MG: Changing pattern of headache pointing to cerebral venous thrombosis after lumbar puncture and intravenous highdose corticosteroids. Headache 1999;39:559–564.
85 Wilder-Smith E, Kothbauer-Margreiter I, Lammle B, Sturzenegger M, Ozdoba C, Hauser SP: Dural puncture and activated protein C resistance: risk factors for cerebral venous sinus thrombosis. J Neurol Neurosurg Psychiatry 1997;63:351–356.
86 Stephens PH, Lennox G, Hirsch N, Miller D: Superior sagittal sinus thrombosis after internal jugular vein cannulation. Br J Anaesth 1991;67:476–479.
87 Larkey D, Williams CR, Fanning J, Hilgers RD, Graham DR, Fortin CJ: Fatal superior sagittal sinus thrombosis associated with internal jugular vein catheterization. Am J Obstet Gynecol 1993;169:1612–1614.
88 Birdwell BG, Yeager R, Whitsett TL: Pseudotumor cerebri: a complication of catheter-induced subclavian vein thrombosis. Arch Intern Med 1994;154:808–811.
89 Schummer W, Schummer C, Weiller C: Dural sinus thrombosis: a rare but potential deleterious complication of a central venous catheter. Intensive Care Med 2001;27:618–619.
90 Nadkarni TD, Dindorkar KS, Desai K, Goel A: Cavernous sinus thrombosis and air embolism following surgery for acoustic neurinoma: a case report. Neurol India 2002;50:201–203.
91 Garrido E, Fahs GR: Cerebral venous and sagittal sinus thrombosis after transcallosal removal of a colloid cyst of the third ventricle: case report. Neurosurgery 1990;26:540–542.
92 Emir M, Ozisik K, Cagli K, Bakuy V, Ozisik P, Sener E: Dural sinus thrombosis after cardiopulmonary bypass. Perfusion 2004;19:133–135.
93 Wustenberg EG, Offergeld C, Zahnert T, Huttenbrink KB, Kittner T: Extension of intracranial thrombosis after unilateral dissection of the internal jugular vein. Arch Otolaryngol Head Neck Surg 2005;131:430–433.
94 Keiper GL Jr, Sherman JD, Tomsick TA, Tew JM Jr: Dural sinus thrombosis and pseudotumor cerebri: unexpected complications of suboccipital craniotomy and translabyrinthine craniectomy. J Neurosurg 1999;91:192–197.
95 Sebire G, Tabarki B, Saunders DE, Leroy I, Liesner R, Saint-Martin C, Husson B, Williams AN, Wade A, Kirkham FJ: Cerebral venous sinus thrombosis in children: risk factors, presentation, diagnosis and outcome. Brain 2005;128:477–489.
96 Yerby MS, Bailey GM: Superior sagittal sinus thrombosis 10 years after surgery for ulcerative colitis. Stroke 1980;11:294–296.
97 Gates PC: Cerebral venous thrombosis. A retrospective review. Aust N Z J Med 1986;16:766–770.
98 Heller C, Heinecke A, Junker R, Knofler R, Kosch A, Kurnik K, Schobess R, von Eckardstein A, Strater R, Zieger B, Nowak-Gottl U; Childhood Stroke Study Group: Cerebral venous thrombosis in children: a multifactorial origin. Circulation 2003;16:1362–1367.
99 DiNubile MJ: Septic thrombosis of the cavernous sinuses. Arch Neurol 1988;45:567–572.
100 Southwick FS, Richardson EP Jr, Swartz MN: Septic thrombosis of the dural venous sinuses. Medicine (Baltimore)1986;65:82–106.
101 Finsterer J, Kladosek A, Nagelmeier IE, Becherer A, Matula C, Stradal KH, Wolf K, Czech T, Stanek G: Chronic granulomatous meningitis with multiple cranial nerve lesions hydrocephalus, stroke, sinus thrombosis, and epilepsy. South Med J 2000;93:1108–1111.

102 Kakkar N, Banerjee AK, Vasishta RK, Marwaha N, Deodhar SD: Aseptic cerebral venous thrombosis associated with abdominal tuberculosis. Neurol India 2003;51:128–129.
103 Fiorot JA Jr, Felicio AC, Fukujima MM, Rodrigues CA, Morelli VM, Lourenco DM, Prado GF: Tuberculosis: an uncommon cause of cerebral venous thrombosis? Arq Neuropsiquiatr 2005;63: 852–854.
104 Messouak O, Amara B, Benjelloun FZ, Tizniti S, Benjelloun MC, Belahsen MF: Thrombose veineuse cerebrale aseptique et tuberculomes cerebraux compliquant une miliaire tuberculeuse pulmonaire. Rev Neurol (Paris) 2007;163:238–240.
105 Van Dyke DC, Eldadah MK, Bale JF, Kramer M, Alexander R, Smith WL, Olivero W: Mycoplasma pneumoniae-induced cerebral venous thrombosis treated with urokinase. Clin Pediatr (Phila) 1992;31:501–504.
106 Niyasom S, Sithinamsuwan P, Udommongkol C, Suwantamee J: Dural sinus thrombosis in melioidosis: the first case report. J Med Assoc Thai 2006;89:242–247.
107 Jones TH, Bergvall V, Bradshaw JP: Carotid artery stenoses and thrombosis secondary to cavernous sinus thromboses in *Fusobacterium necrophorum* meningitis. Postgrad Med J 1990;66: 747–750.
108 Bader-Meunier B, Pinto G, Tardieu M, Pariente D, Bobin S, Dommergues JP: Mastoiditis, meningitis and venous sinus thrombosis caused by *Fusobacterium necrophorum*. Eur J Pediatr 1994;153: 339–341.
109 Jaremko JL, Kirton A, Brenner JL: A 12 year old girl with pharyngitis, meningitis and sinus venous thrombosis. CMAJ 2003;169:811–812.
110 Inghilleri M, Pedace F, Argenta M, Marchetti P, Antonelli M, Bozzao L, Manfredi M: Thrombosis of cerebral veins dural sinuses after paratyphi. Ital J Neurol Sci 1995;16:257–259.
111 Ruggieri M, Polizzi A, Pavone L, Musumeci S: Thalamic syndrome in children with measles infection and selective, reversible thalamic involvement. Pediatrics 1998;101:112–119.
112 Eidelberg D, Sotrel A, Horoupian DS, Neumann PE, Pumarola-Sune T, Price RW: Thrombotic cerebral vasculopathy associated with herpes zoster. Ann Neurol 1986;19:7–14.
113 Pazos-Anon R, Machado-Costa C, Farto E, Abreu J: Síndrome de Ramsay-Hunt complicado con trombosis venosa cerebral como primera manifestación de infección por VIH-1. Enferm Infecc Microbiol Clin 2007;25:69–70.
114 Pérez S, Casado I, García I, Gómez M, Ramirez JM, Luengo E: Infarto hemorrágico por trombosis del seno transverso como complicación de la cirrosis. Rev Neurol 1999;29:1355.
115 Kesler A, Pomeranz IS, Huberman M, Novis B, Kott E: Cerebral venous thrombosis and chronic active hepatitis as part of the antiphospholipid syndrome. Postgrad Med J 1996;72:690–692.
116 Felicio AC, Fukujima MM, Fiorot JA Jr, do Prado GF, de Carvalho Filho RJ, Rodrigues CA, Morelli VM, Lourenco DM: Cerebral venous thrombosis and hepatitis: case report. Arq Neuropsiquiatr 2006;64:1041–1042.
117 Doberson MJ, Kleinschmidt-DeMasters BK: Superior sagittal sinus thrombosis in a patient with acquired immunodeficiency syndrome. Arch Pathol Lab Med 1994;118:844–846.
118 Pedraza S, Rovira A, Saballs M, Capdevila JA: Trombosis de seno longitudinal superior en un paciente con SIDA. Revision de la literature. Rev Neurol 1997;25:247–249.
119 Meyohas MC, Roullet E, Rouzioux C, Aymard A, Pelosse B, Eliasceiwicz M, Frottier J: Cerebral venous thrombosis and dual primary infection with human immunodeficiency virus and cytomegalovirus. J Neurol Neurosurg Psychiatry 1989;52:1010–1011.
120 Turhan V, Senol MG, Sonmez G, Oncul O, Cavuslu S, Tanridag O: Cerebral venous thrombosis as a complication of leptospirosis. J Infect 2006;53:247–249.
121 el Alaoui Faris M, Birouk N, Slassi I, Jiddane M, Chkili T: Thrombose du sinus longitudinal superieur et osteite cranienne syphilitique. Rev Neurol (Paris) 1992;148:783–785.
122 Keuter EJ, Willemse J: The syndrome of acute cerebral thrombophlebitis in a case of malignant malaria. Psychiatr Neurol Neurochir 1963;66:357–361.
123 Krishnan A, Karnad DR, Limaye U, Siddharth W: Cerebral venous and dural sinus thrombosis in severe falciparum malaria. J Infect 2004;48:86–90.
124 Evans RW, Pattern BM: Trichinosis associated with superior sagittal sinus thrombosis. Ann Neurol 1982;11:216–217.
125 el Koussa S, Chemaly R, Fabre-Bou Abboud V, Tamraz J, Haddad N: Trichinose et occlusions sino-veineuses cerebrales. Rev Neurol (Paris) 1994;150:464–466.

126 Macdonald RL, Findlay JM, Tator CH: Sphenoethmoidal sinusitis complicated by cavernous sinus thrombosis and pontocerebellar infarction. Can J Neurol Sci 1988;15:310–313.
127 Van Johnson E, Kline LB, Julian BA, Garcia JH: Bilateral cavernous sinus thrombosis due to mucormycosis. Arch Ophthalmol 1988;106:1089–1092.
128 Mnif N, Hmaied E, Oueslati S, Rajhi H, Hamza R, Marrakchi M, Kaffel N, Kooli H, Ben Salah M, Ferjaoui M: L'imagerie dans la mucormycose rhinocerebrale. J Radiol 2005;86:1017–1020.
129 Sekhar LN, Dujovny M, Rao GR: Carotid-cavernous sinus thrombosis caused by *Aspergillus fumigatus*. Case report. J Neurosurg 1980;52:120–125.
130 Dyken ME, Biller J, Yuh WT, Fincham R, Moore SA, Justin E: Carotid-cavernous sinus thrombosis caused by *Aspergillus fumigatus*: magnetic resonance imaging with pathologic correlation–a case report. Angiology 1990;41:652–657. Erratum in: Angiology 1991;42:172.
131 Breadmore R, Desmond P, Opeskin K: Intracranial aspergillosis producing cavernous sinus syndrome and rupture of internal carotid artery. Australas Radiol 1994;38:72–75.
132 Chandra S, Goyal M, Mishra NK, Gaikwad SB: Invasive aspergillosis presenting as a cavernous sinus mass in immuno competent individuals: report of 3 cases. Neuroradiology 2000;42:108–111.
133 Urculo E, Aranzadi MJ, Ruiz I, Villanua J: Aspergillus granuloma of the cavernous sinus: magnetic resonance imaging with pathologic correlation. Acta Neurochir (Wien) 2005;147:341–342.
134 Deveze A, Facon F, Latil G, Moulin G, Payan-Cassin H, Dessi P: Cavernous sinus thrombosis secondary to non-invasive sphenoid aspergillosis. Rhinology 2005;43:152–155.
135 Kleinschmidt-DeMasters BK, Mazowiecki M, Bonds LA, Cohn DL, Wilson ML: Coccidioidomycosis meningitis with massive dural and cerebral venous thrombosis and tissue arthroconidia. Arch Pathol Lab Med 2000;124:310–314.
136 Raizer JJ, DeAngelis LM: Cerebral sinus thrombosis diagnosed by MRI and MR venography in cancer patients. Neurology 2000;54:1222–1226.
137 Mones RJ: Increased intracranial pressure due to metastatic disease of venous sinuses. A report of six cases. Neurology 1965;15:1000–1007.
138 Brown MT, Friedman HS, Oakes WJ, Boyko OB, Schold SC Jr: Sagittal sinus thrombosis and leptomeningeal medulloblastoma. Neurology 1991;41:455–456.
139 Wester K, Mork S, Smievoll AI: Neuroblastoma and venous sinus thrombosis in an adult patient. Br J Neurosurg 1997;11:241–244.
140 Sigsbee B, Deck MD, Posner JB: Nonmetastatic superior sagittal sinus thrombosis complicating systemic cancer. Neurology 1979;29:139–146.
141 Hickey WF, Garnick MB, Henderson IC, Dawson DM: Primary cerebral venous thrombosis in patients with cancer – a rarely diagnosed paraneoplastic syndrome. Report of three cases and review of the literature. Am J Med 1982;73:740–750.
142 Preter M, Tzourio C, Ameri A, Bousser MG: Long-term prognosis in cerebral venous thrombosis. follow-up of 77 patients. Stroke 1996;27:243–246.
143 Astudillo L, Lacroix-Triki M, Cousin F, Chevreau C: Un syndrome paraneoplasique rare: la thrombose veineuse cerebrale. Rev Med Interne 2007 [Epub ahead of print].
144 Gironell A, Marti-Fabregas J, Bello J, Avila A: Non-Hodgkin's lymphoma as a new cause of non-thrombotic superior sagittal sinus occlusion. J Neurol Neurosurg Psychiatry 1997;63:121–122.
145 McCully KS: Vascular pathology of homocysteinemia: implications for the pathogenesis of arteriosclerosis. Am J Pathol 1969;56:111–128.
146 Ray JG: Meta-analysis of hyperhomocysteinemia as a risk factor for venous thromboembolic disease. Arch Intern Med 1998;158:2101–2106.
147 Den Heijer M, Lewington S, Clarke R: Homocysteine, MTHFR and risk of venous thrombosis: a meta-analysis of published epidemiological studies. J Thromb Haemost 2005;3:292–299.
148 Martinelli I, Battaglioli T, Pedotti P, Cattaneo M, Mannucci PM: Hyperhomocysteinemia in cerebral vein thrombosis. Blood 2003;102:1363–1366.
149 Boncoraglio G, Carriero MR, Chiapparini L, Ciceri E, Ciusani E, Erbetta A, Parati EA: Hyperhomocysteinemia and other thrombophilic risk factors in 26 patients with cerebral venous thrombosis. Eur J Neurol 2004;11:405–409.
150 Cantu C, Alonso E, Jara A, Martinez L, Rios C, Fernandez Mde L, Garcia I, Barinagarrementeria F: Hyperhomocysteinemia, low folate and vitamin B12 concentrations, and methylene tetrahydrofolate reductase mutation in cerebral venous thrombosis. Stroke 2004;35:1790–1794.

151 Ventura P, Cobelli M, Marietta M, Panini R, Rosa MC, Salvioli G: Hyperhomocysteinemia and other newly recognized inherited coagulation disorders (factor V Leiden and prothrombin gene mutation) in patients with idiopathic cerebral vein thrombosis. Cerebrovasc Dis 2004;17: 153–159.
152 Undas A, Brozek J, Szczeklik A: Homocysteine and thrombosis: from basic science to clinical evidence. Thromb Haemost 2005;94:907–915.
153 Ray JG, Kearon C, Yi Q, Sheridan P, Lonn E; Heart Outcomes Prevention Evaluation 2 (HOPE-2) Investigators: Homocysteine-lowering therapy and risk for venous thromboembolism: a randomized trial. Ann Intern Med 2007;146:761–767.
154 den Heijer M, Willems HP, Blom HJ, Gerrits WB, Cattaneo M, Eichinger S, Rosendaal FR, Bos GM: Homocysteine lowering by B vitamins and the secondary prevention of deep vein thrombosis and pulmonary embolism: A randomized, placebo-controlled, double-blind trial. Blood 2007;109:139–144.
155 Barthelemy M, Bousser MG, Jacobs C: Thrombose veineuse cerebrale au cours d'un syndrome nephrotique. Nouv Presse Med 1980;9:367–369.
156 Lau SO, Bock GH, Edson JR, Michael AF: Sagittal sinus thrombosis in the nephrotic syndrome. J Pediatr 1980;97:948–950.
157 Fluss J, Geary D, deVeber G: Cerebral sinovenous thrombosis and idiopathic nephrotic syndrome in childhood: report of four new cases and review of the literature. Eur J Pediatr 2006;165:709–716.
158 Laversuch CJ, Brown MM, Clifton A, Bourke BE: Cerebral venous thrombosis and acquired protein S deficiency: an uncommon cause of headache in systemic lupus erythematosus. Br J Rheumatol 1995;34:572–575.
159 Nishi H, Abe A, Kita A, Toki T, Noda N, Tsuchihashi D, Abe T, Umezu M, Yokozaki H, Fukagawa M: Cerebral venous thrombosis in adult nephrotic syndrome due to systemic amyloidosis. Clin Nephrol 2006;65:61–64.
160 Afsari K, Frank J, Vaksman Y, Nguyen TV: Intracranial venous sinus thrombosis complicating AIDS-associated nephropathy. AIDS Read 2003;13:143–148.
161 Wechsler B, Vidailhet M, Piette JC, Bousser MG, Dell Isola B, Bletry O, Godeau P: Cerebral venous thrombosis in Behcet's disease: clinical study and long-term follow-up of 25 cases. Neurology 1992;42:614–618.
162 Daif A, Awada A, al-Rajeh S, Abduljabbar M, al Tahan AR, Obeid T, Malibary T: Cerebral venous thrombosis in adults: a study of 40 cases from Saudi Arabia. Stroke 1995;26:1193–1195.
163 Vidailhet M, Piette JC, Wechsler B, Bousser MG, Brunet P: Cerebral venous thrombosis in systemic lupus erythematosus. Stroke 1990;21:1226–1231.
164 Finsterer J, Artner C, Kladosek A, Kalchmayr R, Redtenbacher S: Cavernous sinus syndrome due to vaccination-induced giant cell arteritis. Arch Intern Med 2001;161:1008–1009.
165 Mickle JP, McLennan JE, Lidden CW: Cortical vein thrombosis in Wegener's granulomatosis. Case report. J Neurosurg 1977;46:248–251.
166 Konate A, Le Falher G, Crozat-Grosleron S, Riviere S, Le Quellec A: Incidence et presentation des manifestations neurologiques centrales au cours de la granulomatose de Wegener: analyse monocentrique d'une serie de 14 malades. Rev Med Interne 2004;25:183–188.
167 Urban E, Jabbari B, Robles H: Concurrent cerebral venous sinus thrombosis and myeloradiculopathy in Sjogren's syndrome. Neurology 1994;44:554–556.
168 Zhang Z, Long J, Li W: Cerebral venous sinus thrombosis: a clinical study of 23 cases. Chin Med J (Engl) 2000;113:1043–1045.
169 Teresa Sartori M, Briani C, Munari M, Amista P, Pagnan A, Zampieri P: Cerebral venous thrombosis as a rare onset of Churg-Strauss syndrome. Thromb Haemost 2006;96:90–92.
170 Harrison MJ, Truelove SC: Cerebral venous thrombosis as a complication of ulcerative colitis. Am J Dig Dis 1967;12:1025–1028.
171 Borda IT, Southern RF, Brown WF: Cerebral venous thrombosis in ulcerative colitis. Gastroenterology 1973;64:116–119.
172 Rousseau B, Belanger C, Lacoursiere Y, Bergeron MG, Saab M, Poncelet P: Colite ulceruse et thrombose veineuse cerebrale. Union Med Can 1975;104:414–417.
173 Sigsbee B, Rottenberg DA: Sagittal sinus thrombosis as a complication of regional enteritis. Ann Neurol 1978;3:450–452.

174 Averback P: Primary cerebral venous thrombosis in young adults: the diverse manifestations of an underrecognized disease. Ann Neurol 1978;3:81–86.
175 Talbot RW, Heppell J, Dozois RR, Beart RW Jr: Vascular complications of inflammatory bowel disease. Mayo Clin Proc 1986;61:140–145.
176 Yerby MS, Bailey GM: Superior sagittal sinus thrombosis 10 years after surgery for ulcerative colitis. Stroke 1980;11:294–296.
177 Umit H, Asil T, Celik Y, Tezel A, Dokmeci G, Tuncbilek N, Utku U, Soylu AR: Cerebral sinus thrombosis in patients with inflammatory bowel disease: a case report. World J Gastroenterol 2005;11:5404–5407.
178 Byrne JV, Lawton CA: Meningeal sarcoidosis causing intracranial hypertension secondary to dural sinus thrombosis. Br J Radiol 1983;56:755–757.
179 Akova YA, Kansu T, Duman S: Pseudotumor cerebri secondary to dural sinus thrombosis in neurosarcoidosis. J Clin Neuroophthalmol 1993;13:188–189.
180 Squizzato A, Gerdes VE, Brandjes DP, Buller HR, Stam J: Thyroid diseases and cerebrovascular disease. Stroke 2005;36:2302–2310.
181 Keane S, Gallagher A, Ackroyd S, McShane MA, Edge JA: Cerebral venous thrombosis during diabetic ketoacidosis. Arch Dis Child 2002;86:204–205.
182 De Keyzer K, Paemeleire K, De Clerck M, Peeters D, De Reuck JL: Diabetic ketoacidosis presenting as a cerebral venous thrombosis. Acta Neurol Belg 2004;104:117–120.
183 Sasiadek MJ, Sosnowska-Pacuszko D, Zielinska M, Turek T: Cerebral venous thrombosis as a first presentation of diabetes. Pediatr Neurol 2006;35:135–138.
184 Fujimaki T, Matsutani M, Asai A, Kohno T, Koike M: Cerebral venous thrombosis due to high-altitude polycythemia. Case report. J Neurosurg 1986;64:148–150.
185 Johnson RV, Kaplan SR, Blailock ZR: Cerebral venous thrombosis in paroxysmal nocturnal hemoglobinuria: Marchiafava-Micheli syndrome. Neurology 1970;20:681–686.
186 Rothman SM, Fulling KH, Nelson JS: Sickle cell anemia and central nervous system infarction: a neuropathological study. Ann Neurol 1986;20:684–690.
187 Feldenzer JA, Bueche MJ, Venes JL, Gebarski SS: Superior sagittal sinus thrombosis with infarction in sickle cell trait. Stroke 1987;18:656–660.
188 Oguz M, Aksungur EH, Soyupak SK, Yildirim AU: Vein of Galen and sinus thrombosis with bilateral thalamic infarcts in sickle cell anaemia: CT follow-up and angiographic demonstration. Neuroradiology 1994;36:155–156.
189 Di Roio C, Jourdan C, Terrier A, Artru F: Drepanocytose et thrombose des veines cerebrales internes. Ann Fr Anesth Reanim 1997;16:967–969.
190 Ciurea SO, Thulborn KR, Gowhari M: Dural venous sinus thrombosis in a patient with sickle cell disease: case report and literature review. Am J Hematol 2006;8:290–293.
191 Cardenas D, Ovbiagele B: Arterial dissection and cerebral venous thrombosis in sickle cell trait. Br J Hosp Med (Lond) 2006;67:380–381.
192 Schulman H, Hertzog L, Zirkin H, Hertzanu Y: Cerebral sinovenous thrombosis in the idiopathic hypereosinophilic syndrome in childhood. Pediatr Radiol 1999;29:595–597.
193 Murphy MF, Clarke CR, Brearley RL: Superior sagittal sinus thrombosis and essential thrombocythaemia. Br Med J 1983;287:1344.
194 Mitchell D, Fisher J, Irving D, Gazzard BG, Guiloff RJ: Lateral sinus thrombosis and intracranial hypertension in essential thrombocythaemia. J Neurol Neurosurg Psychiatry 1986;49:218–219.
195 Stolz E, Valdueza JM, Grebe M, Schlachetzki F, Schmitt E, Madlener K, Rahimi A, Kempkes-Matthes B, Blaes F, Gerriets T, Kaps M: Anemia as a risk factor for cerebral venous thrombosis? An old hypothesis revisited: results of a prospective study. J Neurol 2007;254:729–734.
196 deVeber G, Andrew M: Cerebral sinovenous thrombosis in children. N Engl J Med 2001;345:417–423.
197 Wermes C, Fleischhack G, Junker R, Schobess R, Schwabe D, Sykora KW, Nowak-Gottl U: Cerebral venous sinus thrombosis in children with acute lymphoblastic leukemia carrying the MTHFR TT677 genotype and further prothrombotic risk factors. Klin Padiatr 1999;211:211–214.
198 Gonzalez JL, Posada I, Ramo C, Calandre L: Trombosis venosa cerebral como complicacion del tratamiento de la leucemia linfoblastica aguda-T con L-asparaginasa. Med Clin (Barc) 1986;87:566.

199 Tomura N, Sashi R, Hashimoto M, Hirano H, Sato K, Hirano Y, Watarai J, Watanabe A: [MRI abnormalities of the brain in neurologic complications following treatment of cancer in children]. No To Shinkei 1996;48:623–630.

200 Millot F, Traore P, Boinot C, Vandermarcq P, Sadoun A, Brizard A, Guilhot F: Hemianopsie laterale homonyme revelant une thrombophlebite cerebrale: role d'un deficit en proteine S induit par la l-asparaginase. Presse Med 2001;30:855–857.

201 Kieslich M, Porto L, Lanfermann H, Jacobi G, Schwabe D, Bohles H: Cerebrovascular complications of L-asparaginase in the therapy of acute lymphoblastic leukemia. J Pediatr Hematol Oncol 2003;25:484–487.

202 Payne JH, Vora AJ: Thrombosis and acute lymphoblastic leukaemia. Br J Haematol 2007 [Epub ahead of print].

203 Finelli PF, Schauer PK: Cerebral sinus thrombosis with tamoxifen. Neurology 2001;56:1113–1114.

204 Akdal G, Dönmez B, Cakmakei H, Yener GG: A case with cerebral thrombosis receiving tamoxifen treatment. Eur J Neurol 2001;8:723–724.

205 Masjuan J, Pardo J, Callejo JM, Andres MT, Alvarez-Cermeno JC: Tamoxifen: a new risk factor for cerebral sinus thrombosis. Neurology 2004;62:334–335.

206 El Accaoui RN, Shamseddeen WA, Taher AT: Thalidomide and thrombosis: a meta-analysis. Thromb Haemost 2007;97:1031–1036.

207 Pagnoux C, Lutz-Zarrouk V, Michel M, Schaeffer A, Godeau B: Cerebral venous thrombosis in a patient with antiphospholipid syndrome treated with thalidomide. Lupus 2004;13:481–482.

208 Lenz RA, Saver J: Venous sinus thrombosis in a patient taking thalidomide. Cerebrovasc Dis 2004;18:175–177.

209 Shiozawa Z, Yamada H, Mabuchi C, Hotta T, Saito M, Sobue I, Huang YP: Superior sagittal sinus thrombosis associated with androgen therapy for hypoplastic anemia. Ann Neurol 1982; 12:578–580.

210 Jaillard AS, Hommel M, Mallaret M: Venous sinus thrombosis associated with androgens in a healthy young man. Stroke 1994;25:212–213.

211 Sahraian MA, Mottamedi M, Azimi AR, Moghimi B: Androgen-induced cerebral venous sinus thrombosis in a young body builder: case report. BMC Neurol 2004;4:22.

212 Shiozawa Z, Tsunoda S, Noda A, Saito M, Yamada H: Cerebral hemorrhagic infarction associated with anabolic steroid therapy for hypoplastic anemia. Angiology 1986;37:725–730.

213 Hamed LM, Glaser JS, Schatz NJ, Perez TH: Pseudotumor cerebri induced by danazol. Am J Ophthalmol 1989;107:105–110.

214 Chu K, Kang DW, Kim DE, Roh JK: Cerebral venous thrombosis associated with tentorial subdural hematoma during oxymetholone therapy. J Neurol Sci 2001;185:27–30.

215 Guimaraes J, Azevedo E: Phytoestrogens as a risk factor for cerebral sinus thrombosis. Cerebrovasc Dis 2005;20:137–138.

216 Waterstone JJ, Summers BA, Hoskins MC, Berry J, Parsons JH: Ovarian hyperstimulation syndrome and deep cerebral venous thrombosis. Br J Obstet Gynaecol 1992;99:439–440.

217 Aboulghar MA, Mansour RT, Serour GI, Amin YM: Moderate ovarian hyperstimulation syndrome complicated by deep cerebrovascular thrombosis. Hum Reprod 1998;13:2088–2091.

218 Benifla JL, Conard J, Naouri M, Darai E, Bascou V, Neuraz A, Deval B, Guglielmina JN, Crequat J, Madelenat P: Syndrome d'hyperstimulation ovarienne et thrombose. A propos d'un cas de thrombose de la veine jugulaire interne. Revue de la litterature. J Gynecol Obstet Biol Reprod (Paris) 1994;23:778–783.

219 Finelli PF, Carley MD: Cerebral venous thrombosis associated with epoetin alfa therapy. Arch Neurol 2000;57:260–262.

220 Martinez Lage JM, Panizo C, Masdeu J, Rocha E: Cyclist's doping associated with cerebral sinus thrombosis. Neurology 2002;58:665.

221 Meyer-Lindenberg A, Quenzel EM, Bierhoff E, Wolff H, Schindler E, Biniek R: Fatal cerebral venous sinus thrombosis in heparin-induced thrombotic thrombocytopenia. Eur Neurol 1997;37: 191–192.

222 Jacquin V, Salama J, Le Roux G, Delaporte P: Thromboses veineuses cerebrales et des membres superieurs associees a une thrombopenie, induites par le polysulfate de pentosane. Ann Med Interne (Paris) 1988;139:194–197.

223 Rice L, Kennedy D, Veach A: Pentosan induced cerebral sagittal sinus thrombosis: a variant of heparin induced thrombocytopenia. J Urol 1998;160:2148.
224 Hoffman EP, Koo AH: Cerebral thrombosis associated with Amicar therapy. Radiology 1979;131:687–689.
225 Achiron A, Gornish M, Melamed E: Cerebral sinus thrombosis as a potential hazard of antifibrinolytic treatment in menorrhagia. Stroke 1990;21:817–819.
226 Katz KA, Hivnor CM, Geist DE, Shapiro M, Ming ME, Werth VP: Stroke and deep venous thrombosis complicating intravenous immunoglobulin infusions. Arch Dermatol 2003;139:991–993.
227 Eikmeier G, Kuhlmann R, Gastpar M: Thrombosis of cerebral veins following intravenous application of clomipramine. J Neurol Neurosurg Psychiatry 1988;51:1461.
228 Wasay M, Bakshi R, Kojan S, Bobustuc G, Dubey N: Superior sagittal sinus thrombosis due to lithium: local urokinase thrombolysis treatment. Neurology 2000;54:532–533.
229 Rufa A, Cerase A, Monti L, Dotti MT, Giorgio A, Sicurelli F, Federico A: Recurrent venous thrombosis including cerebral venous sinus thrombosis in a patient taking sildenafil for erectile dysfunction. J Neurol Sci 2007 [Epub ahead of print].
230 Rothwell PM, Grant R: Cerebral venous sinus thrombosis induced by 'ecstasy'. J Neurol Neurosurg Psychiatry 1993;56:1035.
231 Krausz MM, Feinsod M, Beller AJ: Bilateral transverse sinus obstruction in benign intracranial hypertension due to hypervitaminosis A. Isr J Med Sci 1978;14:858–861.
232 Deschiens MA, Conard J, Horellou MH, Ameri A, Preter M, Chedru F, Samana MM, Bousser MG: Coagulation studies, factor V Leiden, and anticardiolipin antibodies in 40 cases of cerebral venous thrombosis. Stroke 1996;27:1724–1730.
233 Ergan M, Hansen von Bunau F, Courtheoux P, Viader F, Prouzeau S, Marcelli C: Cerebral vein thrombosis after an intrathecal glucocorticoid injection. Rev Rhum Engl Ed 1997;64:513–516.
234 Milhaud D, Heroum C, Charif M, Saulnier P, Pages M, Blard JM: Dural puncture and corticotherapy as risk factors for cerebral venous sinus thrombosis. Eur J Neurol 2000;7:123–124.
235 Stolz E, Klotzsch C, Schlachetzki F, Rahimi A: High-dose corticosteroid treatment is associated with an increased risk of developing cerebral venous thrombosis. Eur Neurol 2003;49:247–248.
236 Barron TF, Gusnard DA, Zimmerman RA, Clancy RR: Cerebral venous thrombosis in neonates and children. Pediatr Neurol 1992;8:112–116.
237 Bonduel M, Sciuccati G, Hepner M, Torres AF, Pieroni G, Frontroth JP: Prethrombotic disorders in children with arterial ischemic stroke and sinovenous thrombosis. Arch Neurol 1999;56:967–971.
238 Carvalho KS, Bodensteiner JB, Connolly PJ, Garg BP: Cerebral venous thrombosis in children. J Child Neurol 2000;16:574–580.
239 Huisman TA, Holzmann D, Martin E, Willi UV: Cerebral venous thrombosis in childhood. Eur Radiol 2001;11:1760–1765.
240 de Veber G, Andrew M, Adams C, Bjornson B, Booth F, Buckley DJ, Camfield CS, David M, Humphreys P, Langevin P, MacDonald EA, Gillett J, Meaney B, Shevell M, Sinclair DB, Yager J; the Canadian Pediatric Ischemic Stroke Study Group: The epidemiology and outcome of sinovenous thrombosis in pediatric patients. N Engl J Med 2001;345:417–423.
241 Johnson MC, Parkerson N, Ward S, de Alarcon PA: Pediatric sinovenous thrombosis. J Pediatr Hematol Oncol 2003;25:312–315.
242 Kenet G, Waldman D, Lubetsky A, Kornbrut N, Khalil A, Koren A, Wolach B, Fattal A, Kapelushnik J, Tamary H, Yacobovitch J, Raveh E, Revel-Vilk S, Toren A, Brenner B: Paediatric cerebral sinus vein thrombosis: a multi-center, case-controlled study. Thromb Haemost 2004;92:713–718.
243 Shevell MI, Silver K, O'Gorman AM, Watters GV, Montes JL: Neonatal dural sinus thrombosis. Pediatr Neurol 1989;5:161–165.
244 Rivkin M, Anderson M, Kaye E: Neonatal idiopathic cerebral venous thrombosis: an unrecognized cause of transient seizures or lethargy. Ann Neurol 1992;32:51–56.
245 Wu YW, Miller SP, Chin K, Collins AE, Lomeli SC, Chuang NA, Barkovich AJ, Ferriero DM: Multiple risk factors in neonatal sinovenous thrombosis. Neurology 2002;59:438–440.
246 Fitzgerald KC, Williams LS, Garg BP, Carvalho KS, Golomb MR: Cerebral sinovenous thrombosis in the neonate. Arch Neurol 2006;63:405–409.
247 Enevoldson TP, Russell RW: Cerebral venous thrombosis: new causes for an old syndrome? Q J Med 1990;77:1255–1275.

248 Garcia JH, Williams JP, Tanaka J: Spontaneous thrombosis of deep cerebral veins: a complication of arteriovenous malformation. Stroke 1975;6:164–171.
249 Houser OW, Campbell JK, Campbell RJ, Sundt TM Jr: Arteriovenous malformation affecting the transverse dural venous sinus – an acquired lesion. Mayo Clin Proc 1979;54:651–661.
250 Chaudhary MY, Sachdev VP, Cho SH, Weitzner I Jr, Puljic S, Huang YP: Dural arteriovenous malformation of the major venous sinuses: an acquired lesion. AJNR Am J Neuroradiol 1982;3:13–19.
251 Convers P, Michel D, Brunon J, Sindou M: Fistules arterioveineuses durales de la fosse cerebrale posterieure et thrombose du sinus lateral. Discussion de leurs relations et de leur traitement a propos de deux cas. Neurochirurgie 1986;32:495–500.
252 Murakami M, Tokuda H, Yokota A, Matsuoka S, Tsukamoto Y: Dural arteriovenous fistulas associated with superior sagittal sinus occlusion. Report of two cases. Neurol Med Chir (Tokyo) 1985;25:662–667.
253 Mayberg MR, Zimmerman C: Vein of Galen aneurysm associated with dural AVM and straight sinus thrombosis: case report. J Neurosurg 1988;68:288–291.
254 Tajima Y, Minami N, Okumura H, Miyasaka K, Moriwaka F, Tashiro K: An unusual case of superior sagittal sinus thrombosis accompanied with dural AV fistula. No To Shinkei 1991;43:981–985.
255 Kutluk K, Schumacher M, Mironov A: The role of sinus thrombosis in occipital dural arteriovenous malformations: development and spontaneous closure. Neurochirurgia (Stuttgart) 1991;34:144 –147.
256 Cataltepe O, Berker M, Gurcay O, Erbengi A: An unusual dural arteriovenous fistula in an infant. Neuroradiology 1993;35:394–397.
257 Pierot L, Chiras J, Duyckaerts C, Jason M, Martin N: Intracranial dural arteriovenous fistulas and sinus thrombosis: report of five cases. J Neuroradiol 1993;20:9–18.
258 Koshimae N, Iwanaga H, Imanishi M, Okuchi K, Tokunaga H, Aoki H, Boku E, Tsujimoto M: Dural AVF of the posterior fossa associated with sinus occlusion presenting as intracerebral hemorrhage: case report. No Shinkei Geka 1995;23:163–167.
259 Sugiura Y, Miyamoto T, Takehara S, Sumiya K, Nozaki T: Multiple dural arteriovenous fistulas following extensive sinus thrombosis: a case report. No Shinkei Geka 1996;24:379–383.
260 Iwakawa J, Umehara F, Nishizawa T, Eiraku N, Osame M: Dural arteriovenous fistulas of the posterior fossa associated with lateral sinus thrombosis presenting as progressive visual impairment. Rinsho Shinkeigaku 1996;36:1095–1099.
261 Iwata A, Nakamura K, Nukina N, Kanazawa I, Iwata M: A case of dural arteriovenous fistula accompanied by sinus occlusion: a serial study with CT scan. Rinsho Shinkeigaku 1998;38:133–137.
262 Ozawa T, Miyasaka Y, Tanaka R, Kurata A, Fujii K: Dural-pial arteriovenous malformation after sinus thrombosis. Stroke 1998;29:1721–1724.
263 Witt O, Pereira PL, Tillmann W: Severe cerebral venous sinus thrombosis and dural arteriovenous fistula in an infant with protein S deficiency. Childs Nerv Syst 1999;15:128–130.
264 Phatouros CC, Halbach VV, Dowd CF, Lempert TE, Malek AM, Meyers PM, Higashida RT: Acquired pial arteriovenous fistula following cerebral vein thrombosis. Stroke1999;30:2487–2490.
265 Singh V, Meyers PM, Halbach VH, Gress DR, Higashida RT, Dowd CF, Smith WS: Dural arteriovenous fistula associated with prothrombin gene mutation. J Neuroimaging 2001;11:319–321.
266 Vilela P, Willinsky R, terBrugge K: Dural arteriovenous fistula associated with neoplastic dural sinus thrombosis: two cases. Neuroradiology 2001;43:816–820.
267 Nishio A, Ohata K, Tsuchida K, Tsuyuguchi N, Hara M, Komiyama M, Tsuruno T, Murata T: Dural arteriovenous fistula involving the superior sagittal sinus following sinus thrombosis – case report. Neurol Med Chir (Tokyo) 2002;42:217–220.
268 Tsai LK, Jeng JS, Liu HM, Wang HJ, Yip PK: Intracranial dural arteriovenous fistulas with or without cerebral sinus thrombosis: analysis of 69 patients. J Neurol Neurosurg Psychiatry 2004;75:1639–1641.
269 Malanga GA, Gangemi E: Intracranial venous thrombosis in a patient with multiple sclerosis. Am J Phy Med Rehabil 1994;73:283–285.
270 Al Bunyan M, Ogunniyi A: Incidental cerebral venous thrombosis in a patient with multiple sclerosis. J Neurol Sci 1997;149:191–194.
271 Albucher JF, Vuillemin-Azaïs C, Manelfe C, Clanet M, Guiraud-Chaumeil B, Chollet F: Cerebral thrombophlebitis in three patients with probable multiple sclerosis. Cerebrovasc Dis 1999;9: 298–303.

272 Stadler C, Vuadens P, Dewarrat A, Janzer R, Uske A, Bogousslavsky J: Thrombose veineuse cerebrale apres ponction lombaire et steroides intraveineux chez deux patients souffrant d'une sclerose en plaques. Rev Neurol (Paris) 2000;156:155–159.
273 Gunal DI, Afsar N, Tuncer N, Aktan S: A case of multiple sclerosis with cerebral venous thrombosis: the role of lumbar puncture and high-dose steroids. Eur Neurol 2002;47:57–58.
274 Vandenberghe N, Debouverie M, Anxionnat R, Clavelou P, Bouly S, Weber M: Cerebral venous thrombosis in four patients with multiple sclerosis. Eur J Neurol 2003;10:63–66.
275 Kadayifcilar S, Gedik S, Eldem B, Balaban H, Kansu T: Panuveitis associated with multiple sclerosis complicated by cerebral venous thrombosis. Ocul Immunol Inflamm 2004;12:153–157.
276 Maurelli M, Bergamaschi R, Candeloro E, Todeschini A, Micieli G: Cerebral venous thrombosis and demyelinating diseases: report of a case in a clinically isolated syndrome suggestive of multiple sclerosis onset and review of the literature. Mult Scler 2005;11:242–224.
277 Berroir S, Grabli D, Heran F, Bakouche P, Bousser MG: Cerebral sinus venous thrombosis in two patients with spontaneous intracranial hypotension. Cerebrovasc Dis 2004;17:9–12.
278 Sopelana D, Marcos A, Arroyo R, Gutierrez E, Cuenca R, Vazquez AV, Gonzalez JL, Egido JA: May intracranial hypotension be a cause of venous sinus thrombosis? Eur Neurol 2004;51:113–115.
279 Flemming KD, Link MJ: Spontaneous CSF leak complicated by venous thrombosis and dural arteriovenous fistula. Cephalalgia 2005;25:751–753.
280 Savoiardo M, Armenise S, Spagnolo P, De Simone T, Mandelli ML, Marcone A, Morciano G, Andreula C, Mea E, Leone M, Chiapparini L: Dural sinus thrombosis in spontaneous intracranial hypotension: hypotheses on possible mechanisms. J Neurol 2006;253:1197–1202.
281 Albayram S, Tasmali KM, Gunduz A: Can spontaneous intracranial hypotension cause venous sinus thrombosis? J Headache Pain 2007;8:200–201.
282 Kataoka H, Tanizawa E, Ueno S: Spontaneous intracranial hypotension is associated with a risk of venous sinus thrombosis and subdural hematoma. Cerebrovasc Dis 2007;23:315–317.
283 Goon PK, Lip GY: Arterial disease and venous thromboembolism: a modern paradigm? Thromb Haemost 2006;96:111–112.
284 Prandoni P, Bilora F, Marchiori A, Bernardi E, Petrobelli F, Lensing AW, Prins MH, Girolami A: An association between atherosclerosis and venous thrombosis. N Engl J Med 2003;348:1435–1441.
285 Prandoni P, Ghirarduzzi A, Prins MH, Pengo V, Davidson BL, Sorensen H, Pesavento R, Iotti M, Casiglia E, Iliceto S, Pagnan A, Lensing AW: Venous thromboembolism and the risk of subsequent symptomatic atherosclerosis. J Thromb Haemost 2006;4:1891–1896.
286 Ray JG, Mamdani M, Tsuyuki RT, Anderson DR, Yeo EL, Laupacis A: Use of statins and the subsequent development of deep vein thrombosis. Arch Intern Med 2001;161:1405–1410.
287 Steffen LM, Folsom AR, Cushman M, Jacobs DR Jr, Rosamond WD: Greater fish, fruit, and vegetable intakes are related to lower incidence of venous thromboembolism: the Longitudinal Investigation of Thromboembolism Etiology. Circulation 2007;115:188–195.
288 van Stralen KJ, Blom JW, Doggen CJ, Rosendaal FR: Strenuous sport activities involving the upper extremities increase the risk of venous thrombosis of the arm. J Thromb Haemost 2005;3:2110–2111.
289 Reich LM, Folsom AR, Key NS, Boland LL, Heckbert SR, Rosamond WD, Cushman M: Prospective study of subclinical atherosclerosis as a risk factor for venous thromboembolism. J Thromb Haemost 2006;4:1909–1913.
290 van der Hagen PB, Folsom AR, Jenny NS, Heckbert SR, O'Meara ES, Reich LM, Rosendaal FR, Cushman M: Subclinical atherosclerosis and the risk of future venous thrombosis in the Cardiovascular Health Study. J Thromb Haemost 2006;4:1903–1908.

Gabriel R. de Freitas, MD, PhD
Rua Mário Pederneiras 55, 206-I
Rio de Janeiro, RJ, 22261-020 (Brazil)
Tel. +55 21 2239 4919, Fax +55 21 2246 2793, E-Mail grdefreitas@gmail.com

Caso V, Agnelli G, Paciaroni M (eds): Handbook on Cerebral Venous Thrombosis.
Front Neurol Neurosci. Basel, Karger, 2008, vol 23, pp 55–76

Thrombophilia and Cerebral Vein Thrombosis

Alfonso Iorio[a], *Chris Barnes*[b], *Maria Cristina Vedovati*[a], *Emanuel J. Favaloro*[c]

[a]Stroke Unit and Division of Cardiovascular Medicine, Department of Internal Medicine, University of Perugia, Santa Maria della Misericordia Hospital, Sant' Andrea delle Fratte, Perugia, Italy; [b]Department of Clinical Haematology, Royal Children's Hospital, Parkville, and [c]Diagnostic Haemostasis Laboratory, Department of Haematology, Institute of Clinical Pathology and Medical Research, Westmead Hospital, Westmead, Australia

Abstract

Cerebral venous thrombosis (CVT) is a multifactorial disease. The idiopathic form represents 12.5% of all CVTs and is diagnosed by excluding known risk factors. As for any form of venous thromboembolism, thrombophilia should be suspected in patients with recurrent CVT or less than 45 years of age or positive family history for venous thrombosis or no evident acquired risk factor. A significant number of CVT patients with thrombophilia also presents other predisposing factors. This suggests that both (1) thrombophilia should be sought for in patients with CVT whether a cause is found or not, and (2) the presence of thrombophilia should not deter the search for other potential causes. Laboratory investigation for markers of thrombophilia in patients with CVT may include the identification of various congenital defects (or deficiencies) of natural anticoagulant pathways (factor V Leiden being the most frequent), as well as of acquired markers (such as antiphospholipid antibodies). A diagnostic test should only be performed if its result will affect the subsequent management of the patient (e.g., the duration of treatment aimed at preventing further thrombotic episodes) or of his family members. The aim of this chapter is to review the available evidence regarding the role played by known thrombophilic factors in CVT and to offer practical suggestions for undertaking laboratory investigations in the most appropriate manner. Odds ratios for CVT were found to be 3.38 for factor V Leiden mutation, 9.27 for Prothrombin G20210A mutation, 32 for antiphospholipid syndrome and 4.07 for hyperhomocysteinemia. Some simple but critical rules are finally given to help when testing for thrombophilia.

Copyright © 2008 S. Karger AG, Basel

Laboratory investigation for markers of thrombophilia (i.e. thrombosis risk) may constitute a part of the clinical workup for patients being investigated for cerebral vein thrombosis (CVT). Such assessments may include identification of various congenital defects (or deficiencies) in natural anticoagulants, as well as acquired markers such as antiphospholipid antibodies (aPL). Such investigations are not always straightforward. For example, congenital defects are rare, and so testing for these needs to be balanced against the high risk of a false-positive diagnosis. Overall, testing should only be undertaken if it will guide future management of the affected patient or other possible family members. Unfortunately, for thrombosis risk, this is by all means not always clear. The aim of this chapter is to review the available evidence regarding the role played by known thrombophilic factors and to offer practical suggestions for undertaking laboratory investigations in an appropriate manner.

Basic Concepts about Thrombophilia

Congenital Thrombophilia

Familial thrombophilia may be defined as a heightened propensity to, or increased risk of, thrombosis that has a familial or genetic basis. Certain factors, or markers, are associated with an increased risk of familial thrombosis, including congenital deficiencies in various natural anticoagulants such as antithrombin (AT), protein C (PC), and protein S (PS) [1–3]. In addition, genetic polymorphisms such as prothrombin G20210A are also associated with thrombosis, as are cleavage-resistant genetic variants of factor V (FV) including FV Leiden (FVL), and which give rise to a condition commonly known as activated PC resistance (APC-R) [1–5]. Each of the above risk factors constitutes an element of increased thrombotic risk, which is compounded when concomitant [1] (table 1). For example, the heterozygous deficiency of AT, PC, or PS, or the presence of heterozygous FVL is thought to increase the relative risk of venous thromboembolism (VTE) by a factor of around 5–10. However, compound defects (i.e. two or more separate risk factors or homozygous FVL) are thought to increase the relative risk 50- to 80-fold.

Acquired Thrombophilia

Acquired thrombophilia (i.e. nonfamilial or genetically based) arises in a variety of situations, which include pregnancy and puerperium, surgery, cancer, immobilization, hospitalization, oral contraceptives (OC), hormone replacement therapy, medication, and aPL. Although only the last in this list can be assessed by laboratory testing, all of these may be considered as risk factors for thrombosis, and assessment additionally included when undertaking clinical

Table 1. Summary of the most common congenital disorders and acquired conditions associated with thrombosis and for which laboratory testing is easily available

Defect (basis)	Estimates of incidence or prevalence					Problems and limitations associated with laboratory testing
	Controls (general population)	Deep vein thrombosis		Cerebral vein thrombosis		
		Thrombophilia population	Approximate RR of thrombosis, OR	Studied patients	OR for CVT	
AT, PC or PS deficiency (congenital)	<0.5%	<5%	10	AT 4/172 PC 6/172 PS 4/172	AT 2.69 (95% CI 0.66–10.96; p = 0.19); PC 11.10 (95% CI 1.87–66.05; p = 0.009); PS 12.49 (95% CI 1.45–107.29; p = 0.03)	High assay variability (poor assay reproducibility); high risk of false-positive case identification (>likelihood of true positive identification); some risk also of false negatives; PC and PS are vitamin K dependent, so false low results also possible as artefact of VKA; identification of PC or PS deficiency will not generally affect type or duration of therapy

Table 1. (continued)

Defect (basis)	Estimates of incidence or prevalence					Problems and limitations associated with laboratory testing
	Controls (general population)	Deep vein thrombosis		Cerebral vein thrombosis		
		Thrombophilia population	Approximate RR of thrombosis, OR	Studied patients	OR for CVT	
APC-R and/or FVL and/or PT-M (congenital)	~5% Caucasians	20–60% depending on case selection	5 (heterozygous FVL) 50 (homozygous FVL) 3 (heterozygous PT-M) 10 (homozygous PT-M)	FVL 469/3023 PT-M 360/2688	FVL 3.38 (95% CI 2.27–5.05; p = 0.001); PT-M 9.27 (95% CI 5.85–14.67; p = 0.001)	False positive and false negatives occur in ~5% of test cases for APC-R, where result may also be influenced by OAT and heparin therapy; identification of APC-R and/or FVL defect and/or PT-M will not generally affect type or duration of therapy
>APS: aPL and LAC (acquired)	<1%	up to 20% depending on case selection	10	aPL 16/152	aPL 32 (95% CI 4.2–243.8)	LAC more consistently associated with thrombosis than aCL or β_2GPI antibodies; LAC testing potentially affected by OAT or heparin therapy; high assay variability/poor assay reproducibility, false positives and false negatives, transient antibodies, considerable laboratory to laboratory variation

HHcy (either)	unknown (?<1%)	up to 20% depending on case selection	2		HHcy 222/472	HHcy 4.07 (95% CI 2.54–6.52; p = 0.001)	Relatively low relative risk for thrombosis; testing requires specific collection conditions (e.g. fasting and/or methionine loading)
High levels of factors VIII, IX, XI (either)	unknown (?<1%)	up to 20% depending on case selection	2				Low relative risk for thrombosis; testing possibly influenced by OAT and heparin therapy; not always clear what constitutes a 'high' level

aCL = Anticardiolipin antibodies, APC-R = activated protein C deficiency, aPL = antiphospholipid antibodies, APS = antiphospholipid syndrome, AT = antithrombin, $ß_2$GPI = anti $ß_2$ glycoprotein I antibodies, CI = confidence intervals, CVT = cerebral vein thrombosis, FVL = factor V Leiden mutation, Hcy = homocystein, HHcy = hyperhomocysteinemia, LAC = lupus anticoagulant, MTHFR = metylentetrahydrofolate reductase, OAT = oral anticoagulant therapy, OC = oral contraceptives, OR = odds ratio, PC = protein C, PS = protein S, PT-M = prothrombin G20210A mutation, RR = relative risk, VKA = vitamin K antagonists, VTE = venous thromboembolism.

Thrombosis risk is significantly compounded when multiple defects are present. Table represents a synopsis of published data.

reviews or considering possible prophylaxis of thrombosis-prone individuals. Other potential markers of thrombophilia that can be assessed by laboratory testing are hyperhomocysteinemia (HHcy) and high levels of some clotting factors such as factors VIII, IX and XI (table 1). These events may be acquired or inherited.

Thrombophilia and Cerebral Venous Thrombosis

According to published case series, thrombophilia represents up to 34.1% of all causes of CVT, genetic and acquired thrombophilia representing up to 22.4 and 15.7% of cases, respectively [6, 7]. In the following paragraphs, we will review the published evidence of association between CVT and common causes of thrombophilia.

Genetic Thrombophilias

AT, PC and PS Deficiency

Prevalence of AT, PC and PS defects in patients with CVT are 2.5, 5.2 and 3.1% respectively, according to the study of Martinelli et al. [8]. Dentali et al. [9] identified two high quality studies investigating the role of AT, PC, and PS deficiencies as risk factors for CVT [8, 10]. The combined odds ratio (OR) of the 2 studies was 2.69 (95% CI, 0.66–10.96; $p = 0.19$) for AT, 11.10 (95% CI, 1.87–66.05; $p = 0.009$) for PC and 12.49 for PS (95% CI, 1.45–107.29; $p = 0.03$). Moreover, several case reports can be found in the literature of patients with CVT and familial AT deficiency [11, 12], PC deficiency [13–15] and PS deficiency [16, 17]. However, due to the overall low number of patients in all these studies, the confidence interval around the overall mean risk ratio remains very wide, and it is impossible to draw any definite conclusion.

FVL Mutation

Activated PC is the antithrombotic protein that normally cleaves and inactivates coagulation factors Va and VIIIa. In 1993, Dahlback et al. [18] described a new cause of familial thrombophilia characterized by a poor anticoagulant response to APC (APC-R) that was later related to a mutation in the blood coagulation FV gene (Arg506Gln), called FVL [19]. The prevalence of the FVL mutation ranges from 0 to 7% [20] in Caucasians, and the mutation is responsible for 95% of APC-R cases. APC-R and FVL are a major risk factor for VTE, found in about 15–20% of patients [21–24].

A meta-analysis by Dentali et al. [9] (including thirteen studies, 469 case and 3,023 control subjects) found a pooled OR for CVT in patients with FVL mutation of 3.38 (95% CI, 2.27–5.05; $p < 0.001$). Prevalence of FVL has been found in 10–25% of CVT patients in small case-control studies [25–31]. According to Tufano et al. [32], the frequency of the FVL allele was 10% (2/20) in patients with CVT and almost half (5.8%, 19/328) in controls (OR 1.8; 95% CI, 0.39–8.4; $p = 0.34$). Similarly, Ludemann et al. [31] found the presence of heterozygous FVL mutation in 14.5% of patients with CVT but in only 6.25% of controls (RR = 2.55).

Prothrombin Mutation

Prothrombin is a key protein in the process of hemostasis. There are few mutations in the prothrombin gene leading to hypo- or dysprothrombinemia, and recently a mutation with the substitution of G to A at position 20210 has been recognized as the second most common hereditary risk factor for deep venous thrombosis as well as CVT [30, 33–37]. Patients with PT-M have higher levels of plasma prothrombin, but it is supposed that their risk of VTE increases markedly only if other risk factors – mostly acquired, such as smoking and the use of OC – are present [30, 37]. Several case reports of association between PT-M and CVT were published [30, 34–36, 38–45].

The meta-analysis by Dentali et al. [9] found 9 studies investigating the role of PT-M in CVT, for a total of 360 patients and 2,688 controls. The pooled OR for CVT was 9.27 (95% CI, 5.85–14.67; $p < 0.001$) in patients with PT-M compared with controls. Among single studies who found PT-M to be a significant risk factor for CVT [30, 34, 46], Martinelli et al. [30] showed that PT-M increases the risk of CVT by a factor of 10. This relation was not affected by the concomitant presence of the FVL mutation. Rodrigues et al. [46] investigated the prevalence of PT-M in 42 consecutive patients with objectively confirmed diagnosis of CVT and compared them with 134 healthy subjects and found this mutation in 16.7% of patients and 0.7% of the control group, yielding an OR for CVT of 26.6 (95% CI, 3.2–223.5).

Other Congenital Thrombophilic Conditions

Sporadic case reports on the association between CVT and hyperfibrinogenemia or congenital deficiencies in the fibrinolytic pathway (tPA deficiency and plasminogen deficiency) were reported [47]. Mutations of FV other than FVL exist but do not appear to be related to the development of CVT. Dindagur et al. [48] investigated the presence of FV A4070G (R2 allele) in 50 Indian women with puerperal CVT and 100 healthy controls. They found 6 cases (12%) heterozygous (none homozygous) and 12 controls (12%; 9 heterozygous and 3 homozygous) for FV A4070G mutation (OR 1.00; 95% CI, 0.31–3.13, $p = 1.000$). They also did not find co-inheritance of FV A4070G with FV G1691A in any of the subjects and observed that the A4070G mutation in FV is highly prevalent in the Indian population but not associated with an increased risk of CVT in Indian puerperal women.

Acquired Thrombophilia

Antiphospholipid Antibody Syndrome

Antiphospholipid syndrome (APS) is an autoimmune disease characterized by clinical manifestations like venous or arterial thrombosis or pregnancy complications and occurrence of repeatedly elevated levels of antiphospholipid antibodies (generically aPL, most commonly anticardiolipin antibodies, aCL) [49]. The incidence of thrombotic complications in patients with APS is near 2.5% patient/year [50]. Lupus anticoagulant (LAC) is a recognized risk factor for VTE (OR 3.6; 95% CI, 1.2–10.9) in patients with APS [51] and this risk increases to 10 times when LAC is associated with β_2-glycoprotein I (β_2GPI) [52], which is one of the main target antigens of aPL [53]. Several hypotheses have been proposed to explain the mechanisms by which aPL promote thrombosis [54–56], but their discussion falls beyond the boundaries of this paper.

The presence of aPL (aCL or LAC) has been suggested as a risk factor for CVT [6, 57–62]. Most of the reported cases refer to patients with systemic lupus erythematosus, but few cases of CVT associated only with LAC [58, 60, 62] or aCL [25, 58, 61, 63–65] were reported. The prevalence of APS in patients with CVT is reported mainly between 7 to 10% [8, 25, 66]. Two studies evaluated APS as risk factor for CVT. The first [67] evaluated the role of aCL in CVT and found a significantly higher incidence of aCL in patients (7/31) in comparison to controls (1/31) (OR 8.75; 95% CI, 1.01–75.64). The second [8] considered APS patients and found a higher incidence of aPL in patients with CVT (9/121) compared with controls (0/242).

Mixed Thrombophilia

Hyperhomocysteinemia

In general, elevated plasma levels of homocysteine are associated with an increased risk of occlusive arterial vascular disease and VTE. In contrast, little information about the role of homocysteine in CVT is available. HHcy (normal range 5–15 mM) has been reported in 27–43% of patients with CVT according to some authors [8, 68].

A meta-analysis [9] of the 4 case-control studies evaluating HHcy in patients with CVT [8, 68–70] showed a pooled OR of 4.07 (95% CI, 2.54–6.52; $p < 0.001$) for CVT in patients with HHCy.

Martinelli et al. [8] published a case-control study on CVT and HHcy and found that HHcy was present in 33 of 121 patients (27%) and 20 of 242 healthy controls (8%; OR, 4.2; 95% CI, 2.3–7.5). The multivariate analysis including HHcy, serum folate, cobalamin, and the 677CT-*MTHFR* mutation showed that the only variable associated with a heightened risk of cerebral vein thrombosis was HHcy (OR, 5.4; 95% CI, 2.6–11.4). Two years later, Tufano et al. [32] confirmed that the frequency of the 677CT MTHFR genotype was 20% (4/20) in patients with CVT and 18.3% (60/328) in controls (OR 1.1, 95% CI, 0.3–3.2; $p = 0.75$, χ^2 test). Cantu et al. [69] published a case-control study on 45 patients with CVT and found that high plasma concentrations of homocysteine and low plasma folate levels were associated with an increased risk of CVT in a population with low socioeconomic conditions and deficient nutritional status. The authors hypothesized that HHcy may contribute to the relatively high incidence of CVT in the Mexican population (where CVT represent 8% of all cases of cerebrovascular disorders in a Mexican registry [71]). Further, HHcy was found in 13/30 of patients with idiopathic CVT (43.3%) versus 4/40 (10%) of sex-matched healthy controls (OR = 6.88, p = 0.002) [68].

The Relevance of the Association of More Than One Thrombophilic Risk Factor and the Effect of Age, Pregnancy and Other Conditions

Association of Thrombophilic Risk Factors

Even the best planned case control study reported in the previous paragraphs could not specifically evaluate the effect of a single thrombophilic risk factor, since the necessary super-selected population does not permit to get clinically useful confidence intervals. Even more difficult to assess is the combined effect of several thrombophilic factors coexisting in the same patient, although this is an unlikely or rare occurrence. However, in the field of idiopathic venous thrombosis the relative risk point estimate for the combination of thrombophilic risk factors, even if defined by wide confidence intervals, is usually very high [30, 39]. Congenital deficiencies in AT, PC and PS can be associated with FVL [72–74]. The coexistence of PT-M and FVL mutations has already been associated with juvenile and recurrent VTE [39, 75], and the presence of the homozygous MTHFR variant increases the risk of venous thrombosis in FVL carriers [76].

The issue of the value of combined thrombophilic risk factors in the field of CVT was dealt with in some of the previously mentioned papers. Tufano et al. [32] reported the presence of associated mutations in 3 patients (15%): 2 with PT-M mutation plus MTHFR and 1 with PT-M plus FVL, and showed an increased risk for the 3 combinations (OR 5.6; 95% CI, 1.1–25.3; p = 0.03).

Similar associations were also reported by Madonna et al. [77]. In 2005, Le Cam-Duchez et al. [78] retrospectively evaluated that CVT risk is increased in patients with PT-M G20210A mutation when associated with the PC promoter CG haplotype (OR = 19.8; 95% CI, 2.1–186.5).

Pregnancy, Elderly and Other Predisposing Conditions

The majority of the studies already presented also reported cases of association of thrombophilic genes with known triggering factors such as pregnancy, puerperium, estrogen-containing preparations, other systemic diseases. The role of these conditions is treated in more detail elsewhere in this book, but some basic issues are reported here to permit discussion of their role in the interaction with thrombophilic risk factors.

Pregnancy and Related Conditions

Pregnancy, puerperium and the use of estrogen-containing preparations are considered triggering factors for venous thrombosis. Pregnancy induces several changes in coagulation system, which persist at least during early puerperium, resulting in a prothrombotic state. Hypercoagulability worsens further after delivery as a result of volume depletion and trauma and in the case of gravidic hypertension. During puerperium, additional risk factors include caesarean delivery and infections (other than pneumonia or influenza). In the case series of Ferro et al. [6], pregnancy and puerperium are reported in 6.3 and 13.8%, respectively, of the female population with CVT younger than 50 years.

Genetic Thrombophilias

In the series of Deschiens et al. [25] none of the 4 cases with FVL was found in the group of idiopathic CVT patients. All had associated risk factors or potential causes: systemic lupus, postpartum, primary APS, nephrotic syndrome, cervical myelitis. This strongly suggests that either the presence of FVL is coincidental or that other circumstantial risk factors (such as pregnancy or OC) are crucial in the occurrence of CVT in these subjects [27, 79]. Further, Martinelli et al. [8] reported an OR of 79.3 (95% CI, 10.0–629.4) for the combination of PT-M and OC in patients with CVT. The same study also reported data on the association between FVL and OC with an OR of 30.0 (95% CI, 3.4–263.0). In 2005, Le Cam-Duchez et al. [78] retrospectively evaluated that CVT risk is increased in females with PT-M on estrogen treatment (OR = 24; 95% CI, 2.26–127.3). Rodrigues et al. [46] found that 72% of their 42 consecutive patients with CVT had at least one acquired risk factor or predisposing condition for VTE and that of the 7 carriers of PT-M 5 had other known acquired predisposing conditions. Moreover, they found that among the

5 women with inherited thrombophilia, there were 4 who were also OC users. These data stress the importance of looking for APC-R and prothrombin mutation in all patients with CVT, whatever the cause, and even in the absence of personal or family history of venous thrombosis. However, as a caveat to this recommendation, please refer to 'Laboratory Testing for Thrombophilia in CVT Patients' below.

Acquired Thrombophilias

Beside systemic lupus, CVT has occasionally been reported with aCL, but other predisposing factors were also frequently present: pregnancy [58], nephrotic syndrome [58] or postpartum [80]. This suggests that factors other than aCL alone are important to induce CVT. In a case series of 40 CVT patients [25], in 2 of the 3 patients with aCL antibodies other conditions coexisted: systemic lupus and FVL in one, FVL in the other. Seventy-five percent of the aCL patients (6/8) in the study of Carhuapoma et al. [65] were associated with OC use, pregnancy, or puerperium. A similar coexistence of risk factors such as PS deficiency, OC use, or puerperium in patients with peripheral venous thrombosis or CVT carrying the FVL mutation is being recognized with increased frequency [25, 64, 72, 73, 79, 81]. The combination of HHcy and OC increased the risk to an OR of 19.5 (95% CI, 5.7–67.3) in patients with CVT [8].

Age

Age is the strongest risk factor for venous thrombosis. This also applies to CVT. Data from the registry of Ferro et al. [82] evidenced differences between the young and middle-aged population (<65 years) and the elderly population (≥65 years). Statistically significant differences have been found for the idiopathic form (37% in the elderly and 10% in the young and middle-aged), the presence of polycythemia and thrombocythemia (12 vs. 2%, respectively, in the two populations) and the presence of solid neoplasms outside central nervous system (CNS), CNS disorders, or dural fistulae (all more frequent in the elderly). No OC, pregnancy, puerperium and hormone replacement therapy were found in the female population aged ≥65 years. A case series of 123 patients from birth to 18 years [83] showed that the most frequent prothrombotic marker was the presence of aCL. Other abnormalities included decreased levels of PC, AT, PS, fibrinogen, and plasminogen and the presence of LAC, FVL, and PT-M (defects are reported with decreased frequency). The deficiencies of AT, PC, and PS were in many cases caused by an acquired disorder such as liver disease, nephrotic syndrome, or disseminated intravascular coagulation. Procoagulant drugs were given to 14 children: 11 received asparaginase, and 3 received OC.

Laboratory Testing for Thrombophilia in CVT Patients

As shown from the data reported, the pathogenesis of CVT is multifactorial, and a diagnosis of idiopathic CVT is generally made when a thorough diagnostic evaluation does not reveal any potential risk factor. According to the general rules of VTE, inherited thrombophilias should be suspected if a patient has recurrent CVT, is less than 45 years old, has a family history of venous thrombosis or has no apparent acquired risk factor. However, in a number of CVT cases, acquired (aPL) or congenital varieties of thrombophilia (FVL being the most frequent) are almost invariably associated with other predisposing factors. This suggests that (1) these abnormalities should be looked for in patients with CVT whether a cause is found or not, and (2) their presence should not deter the search for other potential causes. The detection of such abnormalities has major practical consequences on the long-term management of patients to prevent further thrombotic episodes [25]. Conditions such as APC-R unrelated or due to the FVL mutation, PT-M and even aCL that further lead to a prothrombotic state should be suspected in the presence or absence of an exogenous factor.

Pros and Cons of Thrombophilia Testing: Practical Issues in Laboratory Practice

Although laboratory testing may be recommended when assessing patients with confirmed thrombosis, it is important to gain an appreciation of current opinion and debate regarding the relative merits of testing for and against various markers of thrombophilia [1–3, 84, 85]. Most hemostasis laboratories can perform thrombophilia tests, and their availability tends to encourage both wanted and unwanted clinical ordering. Indeed, tests for AT, PC, PS, APC-R, FVL, PT-M, aPL, LAC, and clotting factors are now common procedures for most hemostasis laboratories, and clinically ordered testing has become very popular, i.e. Hcy [86, 87]. The 'for testing' case often relates largely to the common availability of these tests, and to possible influences on future treatment or therapy for both the patient and other possibly affected family members. That is, the tests are widely available, any clinician can order them, and they could influence the manner in which patients or their relatives may be managed, so why not request such testing? The 'against testing' case (or possibly very select testing case) relates to the cost of testing, the known laboratory limitations regarding testing, the high likelihood of false-positive identification, and the fact that identification of many of these markers will not ultimately influence clinical management in most cases. So, overall, testing may help sometimes, but often it will not help, and in some cases may actually result in more adverse outcomes than those that would have arisen from not testing.

The case for AT, PC and PS is a good example. These tests are widely available, and now form a high proportion of the workload for most hemostasis laboratories [87]. Although these deficiencies may account for up to 5% of cases of familial thrombophilia, true congenital deficiencies of AT, PC and PS are in fact very rare, and would be present in <0.5% of the general population [1] (table 1). Laboratory testing for these markers is also problematic, with high assay variability (or poor assay reproducibility), both within and between laboratories [87–89]. Also poorly recognized by clinicians is the fact that the normal reference range is generated by testing a limited number of normal individuals, and mathematically calculated to capture only around 95% of the normal population. Thus, we should expect that up to 5% of laboratory tests are going to represent either a false positive or a false negative. This is not such a problem when testing for fairly common defects, but it becomes a huge issue when testing for rare defects, or when undertaking a battery of tests. What this means in practice, for AT, PC and PS for example, is that for every true positive (congenital deficiency) identified, the laboratory testing will generate at the very least the same number of false-positive cases. Indeed, it is generally even worse than this, because of the previously stated assay reproducibility problems, and the fact that PC and PS are vitamin K-dependent factors with plasma levels consequently influenced by oral anticoagulant therapy (OAT). Most people who have had a major thrombotic event are placed on OAT as part of their management. Most of these patients are also tested for AT, PC and PS because they have had a thrombotic event. If they are inappropriately tested when they are on OAT, the chance that they will yield a false low level of PC and/or PS is very high, and so too is the possibility of a false-positive identification. With local personal experience, confirmed by others, around 30% of thrombophilia-based testing is inappropriately requested by clinicians whilst patients are on OAT [86, 87, 90]. Since the identification of PC and/or PS deficiency will not generally alter the immediate patient management therapy, testing is rarely ‘urgent’ nor it is often generally required. The risk of recurrence of thrombosis from PC or PS deficiency is only around 1.4× the risk of patients without apparent thrombophilia [91], so long-term OAT therapy is rarely considered appropriate [91, 92]. Since the risk of recurrence of thrombosis from AT deficiency is somewhat higher, at around 2× the risk of others [91], longer-term OAT therapy may be considered as appropriate [91, 92].

Although APC-R testing is also potentially influenced by OAT [86, 90], the case for test limitations in APC-R and FVL is somewhat different from those noted above for AT, PC and PS. APC-R and FVL are actually fairly common events in the general population (positive in up to 5% of the Caucasian population; table 1), so the comparative relative risk of a false positive is lower than that for AT, PC and PS. However, the very commonality of APC-R and FVL among the general population suggests a low likelihood of thrombosis risk contribution to any new thrombophilic event when found alone. This has been confirmed by a meta-analysis of published data, which showed that the presence of FVL was associated with increased odds of recurrent VTE of only 1.4 [93]. In other words: (a) most people with laboratory-defined APC-R and/or FVL may never go on to having an initial thrombotic event, so detecting APC-R and/or FVL in a patient that has not yet suffered one thrombotic event will not on its own help predict any future occurrence; (b) detecting APC-R and/or FVL in a patient that has suffered a thrombotic event will not necessarily identify APC-R and/or FVL as the cause of that event; (c) the risk for recurrence of a subsequent thrombotic event in an individual with APC-R and/or FVL is not much higher than that in any other individual; (d) an individual patient having had a thrombotic event and found positive for APC-R and/or FVL will not usually be managed or treated any differently to a patient having had a thrombotic event and found to be negative for APC-R and/or FVL. Thus, in general, testing for APC-R and/or FVL is rarely 'urgent' or practically useful (although, in contrast, selective case testing may be useful – see below).

On the other hand, knowledge regarding the possible reasons contributing to a thrombotic event (e.g. AT, PC, PS deficiency, and/or APC-R and/or FVL) may be useful in terms of familial studies and patient feedback, particularly if compound or combinations of defects are found, or if prophylaxis in high-risk situations (e.g. immobilization on long haul flights) is being considered. Accordingly, clinicians need to balance the 'need' to identify true cases of AT, PC and PS deficiency, and/or APC-R and/or FVL (etc.) against the very high risk of a false-positive identification of AT, PC and PS deficiency, and the common chance of identifying APC-R and/or FVL. The main important considerations are appropriate case selection and follow-up confirmation (see below).

The situation for acquired disorders is again somewhat different from that above. Although testing for antiphospholipid antibodies (aPL) is also a common laboratory test request, the main problems relate to high rates of false positives and false negatives, a high level of laboratory to laboratory (or test method) variation, and poor inter-method standardization [88, 94, 95]. Furthermore, the test most consistently associated with thrombosis is the clot-based LAC test [96], but as this is a clot-based test using plasma, there are again problems of testing patients undergoing OAT, as well as heparin therapy. With immunoassay-based tests (i.e. ACL, β_2GPI), the main problems relate to the method- or laboratory-based bias or variability, so that a positive result in one laboratory is often seen as a negative result in another laboratory [94, 95]. Again, strategies for overcoming the limitations of these test systems are provided in the next section.

Recommendations for Laboratory Testing Strategies

There are two main components of a diagnosis of a familial thrombophilia deficiency such as AT, PC, PS, APC-R or FVL. The first step is a proper clinical evaluation, and this requires taking careful and appropriate clinical histories, both personal and familial. The second component is laboratory testing. A diagnosis of familial deficiency requires elements of both, not one or the other. In the context of CVT, case selection becomes very important – if testing is performed on patients with lower level likelihood for disease, the result is more likely to be a false positive. Clinicians must also recognize the importance of not undertaking laboratory testing whilst patients are on OAT, and in some cases heparin therapy, and should never diagnose deficiencies of AT, PC and PS solely on the basis of reported low laboratory test results. For identification of other thrombophilia-associated markers, similar caveats can be imposed. In general, laboratory testing is recommended only when the findings might be considered clinically useful (i.e. will influence management, either primary or secondary prevention or treatment type and duration). Unfortunately, for general thrombophilia-related laboratory testing, it is not always clear when this might be the case. What laboratories and clinicians both need are some simple, clear, evidence-based guidelines on thrombophilia testing. These guidelines should include whom to test, when to test, and what to test. Although such recommendations have been published [97–99], including very detailed consensus-based publications from the USA and UK, there is still some dissension among the experts. A practical summary of our recommended approach is given in table 2. Some general concepts have to be clarified. Testing for familial markers of thrombosis is rarely 'urgent', so careful consideration is required in terms of timing of assessments, as well as the need for assessments. Do not request these tests whilst patients are being treated for an initial thrombosis (i.e. especially do not test for AT, PC, PS, APC-R whilst the patient is on OAT or heparin therapy or just post-event). Instead, the general recommendation is to request these tests some 4–6 weeks after cessation of any anticoagulant therapy. Recognize any detected deficiency/defect (especially of AT, PC and PS, but also APC-R, LAC, aPL) as a possible false-positive finding that requires repeat testing for confirmation. Exclude the possibility of OAT, heparin therapy, vitamin K deficiency and liver disease, and request repeat tests for AT, PC and/or PS some 4–6 weeks after cessation of any therapy. Also recognize the possibility of transient false-positive aPL results, and repeat testing for LAC or other aPL some 6–12 weeks after the first positive result. Although a rarer event, also recognize the possibility of false-negative results, and that any potential deficiency/defect (especially of AT, PC and PS, but also APC-R, LAC, aPL) may not be able to be conclusively excluded unless a repeat test has confirmed this finding. In conclusion, do not request investigations into thrombophilia-based tests unless you recognize the limitations of such testing

Table 2. Testing recommendations for the most common congenital disorders and acquired conditions associated with thrombosis and for which laboratory testing is easily available

	General comments	Testing recommendations/follow-up
Congenital		
General considerations	Only test for these if familial tendency is established or suspected, or if results will influence subsequent management of patient or family members	
AT, PC or PS deficiency	Rare disorders; do not test when patient is on OAT (PC, PS) or heparin therapy (AT) or if vitamin K deficiency suspected (PC, PS)	If initial test result is abnormal (i.e. suggestive of deficiency): exclude OAT, vitamin K deficiency and liver disease, then repeat test (6 weeks after cessation of OAT) for confirmation
APC-R	Relatively common finding; do not test when patient is on heparin therapy or on OAT, or if vitamin K deficiency is suspected	If initial test result is abnormal (i.e. suggestive of APC-R): exclude heparin therapy, OAT, vitamin K deficiency and liver disease, then request FVL testing for confirmation
FVL, PT-M	FVL is comparatively common; genetic testing has significant psychological issues for some patients when abnormal genetic tests are identified; for example, psychological fears regarding significance or effects on potential offspring are often in excess to actual risks	Although rare, false positives and false negatives do occur; provide or ensure availability of genetic counseling
APS (acquired)		
LAC	Clot based test; do not test if patient on heparin therapy or on OAT, or if vitamin K deficiency is suspected; has highest association with thrombosis of all the aPL assays	If initial test result is abnormal (i.e. suggestive of LAC) exclude OAT, vitamin K deficiency and liver disease, then repeat test (6 weeks after cessation of OAT) for confirmation
aCL and β_2GPI antibodies	Immunoassays; considerable laboratory to laboratory or method to method variation	False positives and false negatives; if initial test result is abnormal (i.e. positive), repeat test (8–12 weeks later) for confirmation
Either		
HHcy	Low relative risk for thrombosis	Testing requires specific collection conditions (i.e. fasting and/or methionine loading)
High levels of factors VIII, IX, XI	Low relative risk for thrombosis; do not test when patient is on OAT or heparin therapy	Repeat test for confirmation if required (e.g. if initial test result is low, i.e. suggestive of factor deficiency): exclude

Table 2. (continued)

General comments	Testing recommendations/follow-up
	OAT, vitamin K deficiency and liver disease, then repeat test (6 weeks after cessation of OAT) for confirmation; if result is high, also repeat for confirmation and ask laboratory to test at a lower plasma concentration for better test accuracy

Table 3. Thrombophilia testing – overriding principles [adapted from 3]

Guiding principle	Comments/considerations
In general, laboratory (pathology) testing should only be performed if useful for patient management	Management might include type and duration of therapy or treatment, and patient/family counseling (this may be often overlooked or undermanaged)
Detection of a congenital defect such as AT, PC or PS deficiency has significant implications for the affected individual and other family members	This is true for detection of both true positives and false positives. The identification of genetic-mutation-related defects (abnormalities), in particular, has very striking psychological effects for those involved
Testing for rare congenital disorders in individuals where there is no previous personal or family history is not indicated and may have adverse outcomes	Rare congenital disorders such as AT, PC and PS have a base incidence (general population) of around 0.02–0.3%. False-positive error rates are as high as 2–10%. Therefore, identification of a false-positive result is potentially more likely than identification of a true deficiency
Testing for rare congenital disorders in individuals where there is a previous personal or family history may or may not be helpful	A negative finding will not assure a thrombosis free life. A positive finding will not guarantee a thrombosis later in life. A positive finding may or may not alter the clinical management undertaken
Unwarranted thombophilia testing is inappropriate	Unwarranted testing is a huge waste of health care funding and will also likely result in unnecessary concerns for affected patients and family members
Thrombophilia testing should only be ordered and managed by clinicians who understand the relative strengths and weaknesses of screening, and can manage the consequences of testing	Thrombophilia testing should not be ordered and managed by clinicians that do not understand the limitations of screening. Clinicians also need to understand, manage and counsel patients positively identified with thrombophilia markers
Laboratories undertaking testing should do so responsibly	Utilize the best diagnostic tests and test panels, minimize errors, participate in external quality control programs to continuously assess performance with peers, and provide expert advice (educational role) to clinicians as required

Table 3. (continued)

Guiding principle	Comments/considerations
Any identified laboratory defect should be repeated for confirmation	Repeat confirmation to exclude a false positive is an important step in patient management
Any identified laboratory defect confirmed by repeat testing should be appropriately followed up by clinicians	This might include referring to, or discussing with, specialist clinicians and genetic counselors

and are able to offer counseling services, or referral to such services, especially in the case of genetic testing. Some additional general principles regarding thrombophilia testing are provided in table 3.

References

1 Mannucci PM: Laboratory detection of inherited thrombophilia: a historical perspective. Semin Thromb Hemost 2005;31:5–10.
2 Tripodi A: A review of the clinical and diagnostic utility of laboratory tests for the detection of congenital thrombophilia. Semin Thromb Hemost 2005;31:25–32.
3 Favaloro EJ: Diagnostic issues in thrombophilia: a laboratory scientist's view. Semin Thromb Hemost 2005;31:11–16.
4 Hertzberg MS: Genetic testing for thrombophilia mutations. Semin Thromb Hemost 2005;31: 33–38.
5 Hertzberg M, Neville S, Favaloro E, McDonald D: External quality assurance of DNA testing for thrombophilia mutations. Am J Clin Pathol 2005;123:189–193.
6 Ferro JM, Canhao P, Stam J, Bousser MG, Barinagarrementeria F: Prognosis of cerebral vein and dural sinus thrombosis: results of the International Study on Cerebral Vein and Dural Sinus Thrombosis (ISCVT). Stroke 2004;35:664–670.
7 Allroggen H, Abbott RJ: Cerebral venous sinus thrombosis. Postgrad Med J 2000;76:12–15.
8 Martinelli I, Battaglioli T, Pedotti P, Cattaneo M, Mannucci PM: Hyperhomocysteinemia in cerebral vein thrombosis. Blood 2003;102:1363–1366.
9 Dentali F, Crowther M, Ageno W: Thrombophilic abnormalities, oral contraceptives, and risk of cerebral vein thrombosis: a meta-analysis. Blood 2006;107:2766–2773.
10 Bombeli T, Basic A, Fehr J: Prevalence of hereditary thrombophilia in patients with thrombosis in different venous systems. Am J Hematol 2002;70:126–132.
11 Tuite P, Ahmad F, Grant I, Stewart JD, Carpenter S, Ethier R: Cerebral vein thrombosis due to hereditary antithrombin III deficiency. Can J Neurol Sci 1993;20:158–161.
12 Gerszten PC, Welch WC, Spearman MP, Jungreis CA, Redner RL: Isolated deep cerebral venous thrombosis treated by direct endovascular thrombolysis. Surg Neurol 1997;48:261–266.
13 Kuwahara S, Abe T, Uga S, Mori K: Superior sagittal sinus and cerebral cortical venous thrombosis caused by congenital protein C deficiency – case report. Neurol Med Chir (Tokyo) 2000;40: 645–649.
14 Ibrahim A, Damon G, Teyssier G, Billiemaz K, Rayet I, Tardy B: Heterozygous protein C deficiency: apropos of 2 cases with cerebral venous thrombosis in the neonatal period (in French). Arch Pediatr 2000;7:158–162.
15 Eon B, Aknin P, Brun JP, Saux P, Gouin F: Protein C deficiency and cerebral venous thrombosis in pregnancy. Ann Fr Anesth Reanim 1989;8:137–139.

16 Iranzo A, Domingo P, Cadafalch J, Sambeat MA: Intracranial venous and dural sinus thrombosis due to protein S deficiency in a patient with AIDS. J Neurol Neurosurg Psychiatry 1998; 64:688.
17 Heistinger M, Rumpl E, Illiasch H, et al: Cerebral sinus thrombosis in a patient with hereditary protein S deficiency: case report and review of the literature. Ann Hematol 1992;64: 105–109.
18 Dahlback B, Carlsson M, Svensson PJ: Familial thrombophilia due to a previously unrecognized mechanism characterized by poor anticoagulant response to activated protein C: prediction of a cofactor to activated protein C. Proc Natl Acad Sci USA 1993;90:1004–1008.
19 Bertina RM, Koeleman BP, Koster T, et al: Mutation in blood coagulation factor V associated with resistance to activated protein C. Nature 1994;369:64–67.
20 Rees DC, Cox M, Clegg JB: World distribution of factor V Leiden. Lancet 1995;346:1133–1134.
21 Koster T, Rosendaal FR, de RH, Briet E, Vandenbroucke JP, Bertina RM: Venous thrombosis due to poor anticoagulant response to activated protein C: Leiden Thrombophilia Study. Lancet 1993;342:1503–1506.
22 Svensson PJ, Dahlback B: Resistance to activated protein C as a basis for venous thrombosis. N Engl J Med 1994;330:517–522.
23 Trossaert M, Conard J, Horellou MH, Samaha M, Elalamy I, Samama MM: Resistance to activated protein C in venous thromboembolic complications. Incidence and clinical manifestations. Presse Med 1995;24:209–212.
24 Simioni P, Prandoni P, Lensing AW, et al: The risk of recurrent venous thromboembolism in patients with an Arg506→Gln mutation in the gene for factor V (factor V Leiden). N Engl J Med 1997;336:399–403.
25 Deschiens MA, Conard J, Horellou MH, et al: Coagulation studies, factor V Leiden, and anticardiolipin antibodies in 40 cases of cerebral venous thrombosis. Stroke 1996;27:1724–1730.
26 Zuber M, Toulon P, Marnet L, Mas JL: Factor V Leiden mutation in cerebral venous thrombosis. Stroke 1996;27:1721–1723.
27 Martinelli I, Landi G, Merati G, Cella R, Tosetto A, Mannucci PM: Factor V gene mutation is a risk factor for cerebral venous thrombosis. Thromb Haemost 1996;75:393–394.
28 de Bruijn SF, Stam J, Koopman MM, Vandenbroucke JP: Case-control study of risk of cerebral sinus thrombosis in oral contraceptive users who are carriers of hereditary prothrombotic conditions. The Cerebral Venous Sinus Thrombosis Study Group. BMJ 1998;316:589–592.
29 Weih M, Vetter B, Ziemer S, et al: Increased rate of factor V Leiden mutation in patients with cerebral venous thrombosis. J Neurol 1998;245:149–152.
30 Martinelli I, Sacchi E, Landi G, Taioli E, Duca F, Mannucci PM: High risk of cerebral-vein thrombosis in carriers of a prothrombin-gene mutation and in users of oral contraceptives. N Engl J Med 1998;338:1793–1797.
31 Ludemann P, Nabavi DG, Junker R, et al: Factor V Leiden mutation is a risk factor for cerebral venous thrombosis: a case-control study of 55 patients. Stroke 1998;29:2507–2510.
32 Tufano A, Coppola A, Varricchione N, et al: Predisposing factors in patients with early-onset cerebral vein thrombosis. Thromb Res 2005;115:439–440.
33 Poort SR, Rosendaal FR, Reitsma PH, Bertina RM: A common genetic variation in the 3′-untranslated region of the prothrombin gene is associated with elevated plasma prothrombin levels and an increase in venous thrombosis. Blood 1996;88:3698–3703.
34 Reuner KH, Ruf A, Grau A, et al: Prothrombin gene G20210→A transition is a risk factor for cerebral venous thrombosis. Stroke 1998;29:1765–1769.
35 Biousse V, Conard J, Brouzes C, Horellou MH, Ameri A, Bousser MG: Frequency of the 20210 G→A mutation in the 3′-untranslated region of the prothrombin gene in 35 cases of cerebral venous thrombosis. Stroke 1998;29:1398–1400.
36 Kellett MW, Martin PJ, Enevoldson TP, Brammer C, Toh CM: Cerebral venous sinus thrombosis associated with 20210A mutation of the prothrombin gene. J Neurol Neurosurg Psychiatry 1998;65:611–612.
37 Dahlback B: Blood coagulation. Lancet 2000;355:1627–1632.
38 Bloem BR, van Putten MJ, van der Meer FJ, van Hilten JJ, Bertina RM: Superior sagittal sinus thrombosis in a patient heterozygous for the novel 20210 A allele of the prothrombin gene. Thromb Haemost 1998;79:235.

39 De Stefano V, Paciaroni K, Chiusolo P, et al: Cerebral vein thrombosis not related to use of oral contraceptives in a 7-year-old child carrier of the prothrombin 20210A allele. Thromb Haemost 1999;81:991–992.
40 Eikelboom JW, Ivey L, Ivey J, Baker RI: Familial thrombophilia and the prothrombin 20210A mutation: association with increased thrombin generation and unusual thrombosis. Blood Coagul Fibrinolysis 1999;10:1–5.
41 Longstreth WT Jr, Rosendaal FR, Siscovick DS, et al: Risk of stroke in young women and two prothrombotic mutations: factor V Leiden and prothrombin gene variant (G20210A). Stroke 1998;29: 577–580.
42 Simons PJ, Vanhooren G, Longstreth WT Jr, Colven RM: Cerebral venous thrombosis and the G20210A mutation of factor II. Stroke 2000;31:543–544.
43 van KJ, Leebeek FW, Dippel DW, Gomez GE: Prothrombin gene variant (G20210A) in a patient with cerebral venous sinus thrombosis. Clin Neurol Neurosurg 1999;101:53–55.
44 Weih M, Mehraein S, Valdueza JM, Einhaupl KM, Vetter B, Kulozik AE: Coincidence of factor V Leiden mutation and a mutation in the prothrombin gene at position 20210 in a patient with puerperal cerebral venous thrombosis. Stroke 1998;29:1739–1740.
45 Heckmann JG, Tomandl B, Erbguth F, Neidhardt B, Zingsem H, Neundorfer B: Cerebral vein thrombosis and prothrombin gene (G20210A) mutation. Clin Neurol Neurosurg 2001;103: 191–193.
46 Rodrigues CA, Rocha LK, Morelli VM, Franco RF, Lourenco DM: Prothrombin G20210A mutation, and not factor V Leiden mutation, is a risk factor for cerebral venous thrombosis in Brazilian patients. J Thromb Haemost 2004;2:1211–1212.
47 Baumeister FA, Auberger K, Schneider K: Thrombosis of the deep cerebral veins with excessive bilateral infarction in a premature infant with the thrombogenic 4G/4G genotype of the plasminogen activator inhibitor-1. Eur J Pediatr 2000;159:239–242.
48 Dindagur N, Kruthika-Vinod TP, Christopher R: Factor V gene A4070G mutation and the risk of cerebral veno-sinus thrombosis occurring during puerperium. Thromb Res 2007;119:497–500.
49 Wilson WA, Gharavi AE, Oike T, et al: International statement on preliminary classification criteria for definite antiphospholipid antibody syndrome: report of an international workshop. Arthritis Rheum 1999;42:1309–1311.
50 Finazzi G, Brancaccio V, Moia M, et al: Natural history and risk factors for thrombosis in 360 patients with antiphospholipid antibodies: a four-year prospective study from the Italian Registry. Am J Med 1996;100:530–536.
51 Van der Meer FJ, Koster T, Vandenbroucke JP, Briet E, Rosendaal FR: The Leiden Thrombophilia Study (LETS). Thromb Haemost 1997;78:631–635.
52 De Groot PG, Lutters B, Derksen RH, Lisman T, Meijers JC, Rosendaal FR: Lupus anticoagulants and the risk of a first episode of deep venous thrombosis. J Thromb Haemost 2005;3:1993–1997.
53 Hanly JG: Antiphospholipid syndrome: an overview. CMAJ 2003;168:1675–1682.
54 Meroni PL, Raschi E, Camera M, et al: Endothelial activation by aPL: a potential pathogenetic mechanism for the clinical manifestations of the syndrome. J Autoimmun 2000;15:237–240.
55 Ames PRJ: Antiphospholipid antibodies, thrombosis and atherosclerosis in systemic lupus erythematosus: a unifying 'membrane stress syndrome' hypothesis. Lupus 1994;3:371–377.
56 Kandiah DA, Krilis SA: Beta 2-glycoprotein I. Lupus 1994;3:207–212.
57 Vidailhet M, Piette JC, Wechsler B, Bousser MG, Brunet P: Cerebral venous thrombosis in systemic lupus erythematosus. Stroke 1990;21:1226–1231.
58 Levine SR, Salowich-Palm L, Sawaya KL, et al: IgG anticardiolipin antibody titer >40 GPL and the risk of subsequent thrombo-occlusive events and death. A prospective cohort study. Stroke 1997;28:1660–1665.
59 Provenzale JM, Loganbill HA: Dural sinus thrombosis and venous infarction associated with antiphospholipid antibodies: MR findings. J Comput Assist Tomogr 1994;18:719–723.
60 Mokri B, Jack CR Jr, Petty GW: Pseudotumor syndrome associated with cerebral venous sinus occlusion and antiphospholipid antibodies. Stroke 1993;24:469–472.
61 Khoo KB, Long FL, Tuck RR, Allen RJ, Tymms KE: Cerebral venous thrombosis associated with the primary antiphospholipid syndrome. Resolution with local thrombolytic therapy. Med J Aust 1995;162:30–32.

62 Boggild MD, Sedhev RV, Fraser D, Heron JR: Cerebral venous sinus thrombosis and antiphospholipid antibodies. Postgrad Med J 1995;71:487–489.
63 Kesler A, Pomeranz IS, Huberman M, Novis B, Kott E: Cerebral venous thrombosis and chronic active hepatitis as part of the antiphospholipid syndrome. Postgrad Med J 1996;72:690–692.
64 Ricchieri GL, Pizzolato G, Fabbri M, Patrassi GM, Sartori MT: Cerebral and vein thrombosis, transient protein S deficiency, and anticardiolipin antibodies. Am J Hematol 1996;52:69–70.
65 Carhuapoma JR, Mitsias P, Levine SR: Cerebral venous thrombosis and anticardiolipin antibodies. Stroke 1997;28:2363–2369.
66 Daif A, Awada A, al-Rajeh S, et al: Cerebral venous thrombosis in adults. A study of 40 cases from Saudi Arabia. Stroke 1995;26:1193–1195.
67 Christopher R, Nagaraja D, Dixit NS, Narayanan CP: Anticardiolipin antibodies: a study in cerebral venous thrombosis. Acta Neurol Scand 1999;99:121–124.
68 Ventura P, Cobelli M, Marietta M, Panini R, Rosa MC, Salvioli G: Hyperhomocysteinemia and other newly recognized inherited coagulation disorders (factor V Leiden and prothrombin gene mutation) in patients with idiopathic cerebral vein thrombosis. Cerebrovasc Dis 2004;17: 153–159.
69 Cantu C, Alonso E, Jara A, et al: Hyperhomocysteinemia, low folate and vitamin B_{12} concentrations, and methylene tetrahydrofolate reductase mutation in cerebral venous thrombosis. Stroke 2004;35:1790–1794.
70 Boncoraglio G, Carriero MR, Chiapparini L, et al: Hyperhomocysteinemia and other thrombophilic risk factors in 26 patients with cerebral venous thrombosis. Eur J Neurol 2004;11:405–409.
71 Barinagarrementeria F, Sandoval JL, Arauz A, Amaya L, Cantu C: A hospital stroke register in Mexico City: analysis of 2045 patients. Neurology 1999;52:442.
72 Van Boven HH, Reitsma PH, Rosendaal FR, et al: Factor V Leiden (FV R506Q) in families with inherited antithrombin deficiency. Thromb Haemost 1996;75:417–421.
73 Koeleman BP, Reitsma PH, Allaart CF, Bertina RM: Activated protein C resistance as an additional risk factor for thrombosis in protein C-deficient families. Blood 1994;84:1031–1035.
74 Zoller B, Berntsdotter A, Garcia de FP, Dahlback B: Resistance to activated protein C as an additional genetic risk factor in hereditary deficiency of protein S. Blood 1995;85:3518–3523.
75 Margaglione M, D'Andrea G, Colaizzo D, et al: Coexistence of factor V Leiden and factor II A20210 mutations and recurrent venous thromboembolism. Thromb Haemost 1999;82: 1583–1587.
76 Cattaneo M, Tsai MY, Bucciarelli P, et al: A common mutation in the methylenetetrahydrofolate reductase gene (C677T) increases the risk for deep-vein thrombosis in patients with mutant factor V (factor V:Q506). Arterioscler Thromb Vasc Biol 1997;17:1662–1666.
77 Madonna P, De Stefano V, Coppola A, Albisinni R, Cerbone AM: G20210A PRTH gene mutation and other trombophilic polymorphisms in patients with cerebral vein thrombosis. Stroke 2000;31: 1787–1788.
78 Le Cam-Duchez V, Bagan-Triquenot A, Menard JF, Mihout B, Borg JY: Association of the protein C promoter CG haplotype and the factor II G20210A mutation is a risk factor for cerebral venous thrombosis. Blood Coagul Fibrinolysis 2005;16:495–500.
79 Vandenbroucke JP, Koster T, Briet E, Reitsma PH, Bertina RM, Rosendaal FR: Increased risk of venous thrombosis in oral-contraceptive users who are carriers of factor V Leiden mutation. Lancet 1994;344:1453–1457.
80 Moreb J, Kitchens CS: Acquired functional protein S deficiency, cerebral venous thrombosis, and coumarin skin necrosis in association with antiphospholipid syndrome: report of two cases. Am J Med 1989;87:207–210.
81 Vermylen J, Blockmans D, Spitz B, Deckmyn H: Thrombosis and immune disorders. Clin Haematol 1986;15:393–412.
82 Ferro JM, Canhao P, Bousser MG, Stam J, Barinagarrementeria F: Cerebral vein and dural sinus thrombosis in elderly patients. Stroke 2005;36:1927–1932.
83 deVeber G, Andrew M, Adams C, et al: Cerebral sinovenous thrombosis in children. N Engl J Med 2001;345:417–423.
84 Martinelli I: Pros and cons of thrombophilia testing: pros. J Thromb Haemost 2003;1:410–411.
85 Machin SJ: Pros and cons of thrombophilia testing: cons. J Thromb Haemost 2003;1:412–413.

86 Favaloro EJ, Orsag I, Bukuya M, McDonald D: A 9-year retrospective assessment of laboratory testing for activated protein C resistance: evolution of a novel approach to thrombophilia investigations. Pathology 2002;34:348–355.
87 Favaloro EJ, Soltani S, McDonald J, Grezchnik E, Easton L: Laboratory identification of familial thrombophilia: do the pitfalls exceed the benefits? A reassessment of ABO-blood group, gender, age, and other laboratory parameters on the potential influence on a diagnosis of protein C, protein S, and antithrombin deficiency and the potential high risk of a false positive diagnosis. Lab Hematol 2005;11:174–184.
88 Favaloro EJ, Bonar R, Sioufi J, et al: Multilaboratory testing of thrombophilia: current and past practice in Australasia as assessed through the Royal College of Pathologists of Australasia Quality Assurance Program for Hematology. Semin Thromb Hemost 2005;31:49–58.
89 Favaloro EJ: Learning from peer assessment: the role of the external quality assurance multilaboratory thrombophilia test process. Semin Thromb Hemost 2005;31:85–89.
90 Florell SR, Rodgers GM III: Utilization of testing for activated protein C resistance in a reference laboratory. Am J Clin Pathol 1996;106:248–252.
91 De Stefano V, Simioni P, Rossi E, et al: The risk of recurrent venous thromboembolism in patients with inherited deficiency of natural anticoagulants antithrombin, protein C and protein S. Haematologica 2006;91:695–698.
92 Gallus AS: Management options for thrombophilias. Semin Thromb Hemost 2005;31:118–126.
93 Ho WK, Hankey GJ, Quinlan DJ, Eikelboom JW: Risk of recurrent venous thromboembolism in patients with common thrombophilia: a systematic review. Arch Intern Med 2006;166:729–736.
94 Favaloro EJ, Wong RC, Silvestrini R, McEvoy R, Jovanovich S, Roberts-Thomson P: A multilaboratory peer assessment quality assurance program-based evaluation of anticardiolipin antibody, and beta2-glycoprotein I antibody testing. Semin Thromb Hemost 2005;31:73–84.
95 Favaloro EJ, Wong RC, Jovanovich S, Roberts-Thomson P: A review of beta2-glycoprotein-I antibody testing results from a peer-driven multilaboratory quality assurance program. Am J Clin Pathol 2007;127:441–448.
96 Galli M, Barbui T: Antiphospholipid syndrome: clinical and diagnostic utility of laboratory tests. Semin Thromb Hemost 2005;31:17–24.
97 Walker ID, Greaves M, Preston FE; on behalf of the Haemostasis and Thrombosis Task Force, British Committee for Standards in Haematology: Investigation and management of heritable thrombophilia. Br J Haematol 2001;114:512–528.
98 Van Cott EM, Laposata M, Prins MH: Laboratory evaluation of hypercoagulability with venous or arterial thrombosis. Arch Pathol Lab Med 2002;126:1281–1295.
99 De Stefano V, Rossi E, Paciaroni K, Leone G: Screening for inherited thrombophilia: indications and therapeutic implications. Haematologica 2002;87:1095–1108.

Dr. Alfonso Iorio
Stroke Unit and Division of Cardiovascular Medicine
Department of Internal Medicine, University of Perugia
Santa Maria della Misericordia Hospital
Via Dottori, Sant'Andrea delle Fratte, IT–06126 Perugia (Italy)
Tel. +39 075 578 2309, Fax +39 178 2218 383, E-Mail iorioa@unipg.it

Caso V, Agnelli G, Paciaroni M (eds): Handbook on Cerebral Venous Thrombosis.
Front Neurol Neurosci. Basel, Karger, 2008, vol 23, pp 77–88

Clinical Presentations of Cerebral Vein and Sinus Thrombosis

Maurizio Paciaroni[a], *Francesco Palmerini*[a], *Julien Bogousslavsky*[b]

[a]Stroke Unit and Division of Cardiovascular Medicine, Department of Internal Medicine, University of Perugia, Santa Maria della Misericordia Hospital, Sant' Andrea delle Fratte, Perugia, Italy; [b]Department of Neurology and Neurorehabilitation, Swiss Medical Network, Valmont-Genolier, Glion-sur-Montreux, Switzerland

Abstract

Intracranial venous thrombosis may occur at any time from infancy to old age and its clinical expression varies widely and sometimes it may present without focal signs. The most common symptoms are: headache, vomiting, transient or persistent visual obscuration, focal or generalized seizures, lethargy and coma, while papilledema is a common sign. There may also be alternating focal deficits, hemiparesis or paraparesis, or other focal neurological deficits depending on the location of the venous structures involved. Symptom onset is either acute, subacute or chronic. Even with a severe initial presentation, partial or complete recovery is possible, underlying the importance of early recognition. Antithrombotic treatment must be administered at diagnosis as soon as possible.

Copyright © 2008 S. Karger AG, Basel

Common Clinical Signs, Symptoms and Clinical Syndromes of Cerebral Vein and Sinus Thrombosis

Cerebral venous pathology is significantly less common than arterial pathologies. Symptoms are often aspecific (table 1) and are related to the specifically involved venous structure, to the presence of valid collateral system and to intracranial hypertension. Unlike in arterial stroke, the symptom onset in cerebral venous thrombosis is usually subacute (2 days to 1 month; 50–80%), in some cases it can be acute (2 days or less) and simulate arterial stroke (20–30%). In patients presenting isolated intracranial hypertension, the onset of symptoms can be chronic (more than 2 months; 10–20%) [1]. Occasionally, symptoms can progress over more than 6 months [2]. Even though onset can seldom simulate

Table 1. Signs and symptoms (%) in patients with cerebral venous thrombosis [51]

Signs/symptoms	
Headache	92
Papilledema	45
Motor deficit	42
Sensorial deficit	11
Seizures	37
Delirium	25
Aphasia	18
Stupor/Coma	13
Oculomotor nerve palsy	10
Visual deficit	9
Meningeal signs	5
Hemianopia	4
Cerebellar signs	4
Pulsatile tinnitus	2
Optic ataxia	1
Vertigo	1
Forced deviation of the eyes	1
Neglect	1
Movement disorders	1
Other cranial nerve palsy	1
Syndromes	
Focal syndrome	40
Encephalopathy	31
Isolated intracranial hypertension	29

an arterial stroke, the characteristics of cerebral venous thrombosis usually differ from those of an arterial stroke. Cerebral venous thrombosis has a more progressive development, strong tendency to fluctuate, association with other manifestations of increased intracranial hypertension and seizures. Other differences are: venous cerebral infarct usually does not fit an arterial territory, more often it is bilateral and hemorrhagic transformation of the lesion is quite frequent.

Depending on the location of the thrombosis and the collateral blood flow, and patient's age, the range of clinical symptoms associated with cerebral venous thrombosis is astonishingly varied, and its clinical presentation is extremely variable and unspecific [3]. The most common symptoms and signs are headache and papilledema due to intracranial hypertension, seizures, focal neurological deficits, and altered consciousness. These can be present alone (pure headache, pure seizures, pure intracranial hypertension) or in association. With decreasing frequency, patients present with one of the following clinical syndromes [4]: isolated intracranial hypertension with headache and papillary edema; headache plus focal neurological deficits and focal seizures; isolated cranial nerve lesions with headache; subacute unspecific encephalopathy; sinus cavernous syndrome with chemosis, protrusion bulbi and painful ophthalmoplegia; unusual presentations.

Frequently, these syndromes overlap and, of course, none of the syndromes is specific for cerebral venous thrombosis [5].

Symptoms and Signs of Intracranial Hypertension

Headache is the most common symptom and it is present in up to 80% of all patients. Headache can present as migraine in migraine patients or tension type headache, but it is usually progressive, continuous and refractory to medical treatment [see the chapter by Alberti et al., this vol., pp. 89–95].

Patients affected by cerebral venous thrombosis can present threatened vision, visual obscuration, visual loss and constriction of the visual field [6]. These symptoms can be related to either the presence of cerebral infarct (involving optic radiations or occipital cortex) or to papilledema, due to intracranial hypertension. Papilledema on fundoscopy can be initially evidenced as optic disc swelling, elevating and blurring. Over a few days, retinal essudates, splinter hemorrhages and infarcts can be observed. Papilledema frequency ranges from 45 to 86% in all cerebral venous thrombosis cases [2, 7] but this finding is less common in acute cases. The presence of papilledema, associated with altered consciousness, age older than 33, intracerebral hemorrhage and an involvement of the straight sinus can be predictors of poor outcome [8]. Furthermore, papilledema is commonly associated with other signs of intracranial hypertension such as headache, vomiting and bradycardia. In the absence of treatment, papilledema is known to lead to optic atrophy [9].

Cerebral venous thrombosis can be overlooked when intracranial hypertension is isolated. In a series of patients affected by cerebral venous thrombosis, 37% had intracranial hypertension as the only sign of cerebral venous thrombosis [7]. Cerebral venous thrombosis can be present with all the classical criteria for idiopathic intracranial hypertension, including normal brain computed tomography (CT) with normal cerebrospinal fluid (CSF) content. Then magnetic resonance imaging (MRI), with magnetic resonance venography should be performed, when necessary, also in patients with isolate intracranial hypertension.

Focal Cerebral Symptoms

Seizures can be initial signs of cerebral venous thrombosis. Their frequency has been reported to range from 10 to 60% in published series. Seizures occur more frequently in children (58%) and neonates (71%) [10]. In a consecutive series of patients with cerebral venous thrombosis, early symptomatic seizures were found in 44.3% of all patients while status epilepticus was found to occur in 12.8% of patients [11]. Patients with cerebral venous thrombosis and epileptic seizures are more likely to be admitted to a neurological intensive care unit than those without epileptic seizures. Motor deficit, intracranial hemorrhage, and cortical vein thrombosis are independent predictors of early epileptic seizures [11]. Principal predictors of death in a series of patients affected by cerebral venous thrombosis were: seizures, mental status disturbances, coma (Glasgow Coma Scale <9), deep cerebral venous thrombosis, right-sided hemorrhage and posterior fossa lesions [12]. Seizures are about equally divided between focal and generalized types; the association of both types is very common. Seizures are usually generalized in patients with isolated intracranial hypertension; by contrast, they are common and often partial in patients who have focal deficit. At present, there is no evidence for a prophylactic use of antiepileptic drugs in patients with cerebral venous thrombosis. The antiepileptic treatment should be started when the seizures enter the clinical picture. Seizures are typically difficult to treat and the optimal duration of treatment for patients with seizures is a subject of debate. Prolonged treatment with antiepileptic drugs for 1 year could be reasonable for patients with early seizures and hemorrhagic lesions on CT scan [13; see the chapter by Ferro and Canhão, this vol., pp. 161–171].

Focal neurological deficits such as paresis, dysphasia, visual-spatial disorders, and homonymous hemianopia are inaugural symptoms in 15% of patients affected by cerebral venous thrombosis and they can be observed in up to 50% during the course of the disease. Focal neurological signs are associated with the presence of large cerebral infarct with and without hemorrhagic transformation: these can be located in the Rolandic, frontal-parietal and parietal-occipital regions near the midline or in the posterior temporal area. Bilateral cerebral infarcts with bilateral symptomatology are common and among their focal symptoms the most common is hemiparesis or hemiplegia present in 34–43% [2, 8]. Motor deficits are known to worsen over days and predominantly affect the legs. When onset is abrupt, cerebral venous thrombosis can simulate arterial stroke; chronic cases mimic tumors while subacute cases can mimic brain abscesses. Patients with motor or sensory deficits, associated with parenchymal lesions accompanied by an involvement of sagittal sinus and cortical vein thrombosis tend to have more epileptic seizures [14]. In rare cases, focal neurological deficits are transient and mimic transient ischemic attack [15].

Consciousness disturbance as the initial sign of cerebral venous thrombosis is rare, although it can be present when the thrombosis affects the deep venous system. Patients may be comatose when large unilateral infarcts or hemorrhages compress the diencephalons and brainstem, when thrombosis involves the deep grey matter of the thalamus and corpus striatum, hypothalamus, ventral corpus callosum, medial occipital lobe and the upper part of the cerebellum. Neurological examination reveals severe dysfunction of the diencephalons, with coma, disturbances of eye movements and pupillary reflexes.

Cranial nerve palsies are reported in 12% of all cases of cerebral venous thrombosis. The cranial nerves that have been described to be involved are III, IV, V, VI, VII, VIII, IX, X and XI, and the involvement can be multiple or single. In rare cases, cranial nerve palsies can be the only sign of cerebral venous thrombosis, especially when there is the involvement of the transverse/sigmoid sinus (VI, VII and VIII cranial nerves) [4]. An isolated peripheral facial nerve palsy was described for segmental occlusion of the ipsilateral transverse sinus [16]. Along with other neurological events, involvement of cranial nerves is known from the previous literature; in the case of thrombosis of the petrosal sinuses, it is mainly characterized by a V nerve palsy for the superior sinus and a VI nerve palsy for the inferior one [17, 18]. In patients with lateral sinus thrombosis, diplopia due to VI nerve palsy and signs of V nerve irritation with temporal and retro-orbital pain, it has also long been known as the Gradenigo syndrome, suggesting involvement of the nerves at the petrous apex. The unilateral or bilateral VI cranial nerve involvement can also be due to the intracranial hypertension itself. The involvement of the III, IV, V and VI cranial nerves can be due to the thrombosis of the anterior cavernous sinus. An involvement of the IX, X and XI cranial nerves is possible when the location of the thrombosis is in the posterior cavernous sinus or the internal jugular vein, or the deep venous system or the cerebellar veins. In this latter case, other symptoms due to the involvement of the brainstem, such as limb or gait ataxia and impaired consciousness, may be present.

Neuropsychological deficits such as impaired anterograde memory, dementia, akinetic mutism, and abnormal movements such as athetoid movements and dystonia, can in rare cases be symptoms of deep cerebral venous thrombosis.

Subacute Unspecific Diffuse Encephalopathy

A generalized encephalopatic illness without localizing signs or recognizable features of raised intracranial pressure is another pattern of presentation [1]. A depressed level of consciousness is the most constant finding, varying from drowsiness to deep coma. This type of presentation is extremely misleading. The differential diagnosis includes encephalitis, disseminated intravascular coagulation, marantic endocarditis, metabolic disorders and cerebral vasculitis [19].

Unusual Presentation of Cerebral Vein and Sinus Thrombosis

The progress on the diagnosis of cerebral venous thrombosis, the routine use of MRI, and a better understanding of the disease have made it possible for physicians to identify unusual presentations of cerebral venous thrombosis – confirming that it can be difficult to diagnose, because of its large spectrum of clinical manifestations.

Subarachnoid hemorrhage has been described as the initial presentation of dural sinus thrombosis [20]. In this case report, 4 patients presented severe headache and neuroradiological features initially suggesting subarachnoid hemorrhage with no associated parenchymal bleeding. Digital subtracted angiography evidenced occlusion of intracranial venous sinuses but did not reveal other causes of subarachnoid hemorrhage. All patients improved with anticoagulant therapy. The exact cause of subarachnoid hemorrhage associated with cerebral venous thrombosis is unknown. A hypothesis could be that venous hemorrhagic infarction can be responsible for secondary rupture into subarachnoid spaces and cause subarachnoid hemorrhages. Patients with cerebral venous thrombosis can present with headache of sudden onset, neck stiffness and imaging evidence of subarachnoid hemorrhage simulating a ruptured intracranial aneurysm. Differentiating cerebral venous thrombosis from subarachnoid hemorrhage in these cases may be further complicated as the CSF in patients with cerebral venous thrombosis can be hemorrhagic.

Isolated psychiatric symptoms such as irritability, anxiety, depression, psychosis, delirium and amnesia are known to be the prevailing symptoms of cerebral venous thrombosis. They can be misleading in the postpartum period.

Reversible parkinsonism and MRI diffusion abnormalities [21] have been described as a presenting symptom of cortical venous thrombosis. In this case report, headache, altered level of consciousness and parkinsonism were described as the clinical feature of a thrombosis in the vein of Galen, internal cerebral vein and straight sinus. Diffusion imaging showed hyperintensity in both lentiform nuclei, the right caudate, both thalami and nonspecific foci in the white matter. At 10 days, MRI showed improvement of the thrombosis; diffusion abnormalities were also markedly better. At 6-month follow-up, there were no clinical signs of parkinsonism.

Specific occasional manifestations such as trigeminal neuralgia have been reported in cerebral venous thrombosis. In this case report [22] trigeminal-like neuralgia was associated with intracranial hypertension secondary to thrombosis of the deep cerebral venous system.

Acute visual loss [23], acute micrographia and hypophonia [24], migraine-like phenomena [25], hearing loss [26], ocular flutter (intermittent bursts of conjugate horizontal saccades without intersaccadic interval) [27] and dizziness when eating [28] have been described as the only symptoms of cerebral venous thrombosis.

Spontaneous bilateral ecchymosis is an extremely rare finding which can be associated with cerebral venous thrombosis in adult and neonate patients [29, 30].

Some authors have hypothesized that transient global amnesia may also be caused by cerebral vein thrombosis. Subsequent venous congestion, in fact, can lead to ischemia or induce a spreading depression in the medial temporal lobes [31].

Finally, cerebral venous thrombosis can also be asymptomatic, particularly in the case of lateral sinus thrombosis, which can be observed on a routine CT scan [32].

Topographic Diagnosis

The location of the thrombosis can determine characteristic clinical patterns.

The superior sagittal sinus thrombosis is present in from 72 to 92% [33, 34] of all of cerebral venous thrombosis cases. However, when the thrombosis is restricted to the superior sagittal sinus, its frequency varies from 13 to 55% in all cerebral venous thrombosis cases. At CT scan, 'the dense triangle sign' and the empty delta sign can be detected. Patients can present typical symptoms of isolated intracranial hypertension with headache, foggy vision, visual loss, nausea, vomiting and cranial nerve palsy (this is the main consideration in the differential diagnosis of pseudotumor cerebri). Yet, more frequently, thrombosis of the superior sagittal sinus can lead to deficiency syndromes with cortical signs such as aphasia, hemianopia and neglect. At the same time, superior sagittal sinus thrombosis can produce cranial nerve palsy, hypoesthesia and hemiparesis that normally worsen over time. Focal or generalized seizures can be present especially in neonates and children. These are frequently observed when focal deficits are present. Rarely can isolated psychiatric symptoms such as irritability, anxiety, depression, psychosis, delirium and hallucinations be present that can lead to a misdiagnosis.

Lateral sinus thrombosis is involved in about 10% of the cases. When isolated, it is known to be asymptomatic and headache can be the exclusive symptom. When this type of thrombosis extends to the contiguum sinuses (superior sagittal sinus, deep venous system, superior and inferior sinuses), intracranial hypertension, consciousness disturbance, focal cerebral signs and cranial nerve palsies (IX-X-XI) [2] may be present. When thrombosis extends to the cerebellar vein, patients with isolated headache develop vomiting and limb or gait ataxia. Involvement of cranial nerves (IX, X) can indicate the involvement of the internal jugular vein. At CT scan, lateral sinus can be spontaneously hyperdense. When asymptomatic and restricted to the lateral sinus, it is often hard to differentiate hypoplasia (present in up to 40% in general population) from thrombosis with conventional MRI even by MR angiography, so digital angiography is often needed.

Cortical vein thrombosis is rare (2–5%), usually asymptomatic and difficult to detect at examination (CT scan and MRI), due to the presence of valid collateral vessels and the specifically different pathology of venous infarcts. Cortical vein thrombosis becomes symptomatic when associated with the presence of parenchymal lesions, which usually consist of large cortical infarcts associated with an acute motor deficit predominantly affecting a leg, cortical signs and epileptic seizures. Focal or generalized seizures followed by hemiparesis, aphasia, hemianopia, or other focal neurological dysfunctions, in the absence of signs of increased intracranial pressure such as nausea, vomiting or papilledema, strongly suggest the presence of cortical vein thrombosis. Headache can be present but without associated signs suggesting intracranial hypertension. Neuroimaging (CT, MRI) usually shows an ischemic lesion that does not follow the boundary of arterial territories and often has a hemorrhagic component, without signs of venous sinus thrombosis. The combination of a nonspecific clinical picture with an atypical lesion on cerebral CT scan may favor the diagnosis of cortical venous thrombosis. Furthermore, in a few cases, cortical venous infarcts are mistaken for brain tumors or abscess and diagnosed only at biopsy. Conventional angiography does not evidence arterial occlusion, but may show cortical vein thrombosis related to the infarct, although there can also be nonspecific findings [35]. The parietotemporal region can be frequently involved in relation to parietal or Labbé vein thrombosis. Isolated thrombosis of the vein of Labbé has been rarely reported. The left vein of Labbé has been most often involved [36]. The vein of Labbé drains the lateral temporal lobe and empties the transverse sinus [37]. Thrombosis can cause temporal lobe hemorrhagic infarction, hemorrhage or edema [38].

The thrombosis of the deep venous system [sinus sigmoideus, sinus petrosus inferior and superior, straight sinus, basal vein (vein of Rosenthal), great cerebral vein (vein of Galen)] is less common and represents about 3–8% of cerebral venous thromboses. Occlusion of the deep cerebral veins is the clinically most obscure of the venous syndromes. It is usually characterized by severe dysfunction of the diencephalon such as coma, pupillary abnormalities, ophthalmoplegia, extrapyramidal hypertonia, and papilledema. Because of the peculiarity of anastomotic connections of the deep venous system, only the simultaneous obstruction of the great vein of Galen and basal vein will obstruct venous outflow [39]. Thrombosis of the deep venous system should be strongly suspected in patients presenting with headache, nausea, vomiting, nystagmus, bilateral or alterning paresis, limb or gait ataxia and impaired consciousness. In these cases, bilateral infarcts with or without secondary transformation involving the thalamus, the striatum, the ventral corpus callosum, the medial occipital lobe and the upper part of cerebellum are usually detected at neuroradiological examination. Isolated depression and disorientation due to bilateral thalamic lesions were described [40]. Thrombosis of the deep venous system has a poor outcome; neuropsychological deficits such as impaired anterograde memory, dementia, hemiparesis, akinetic mutism, and abnormal movements as athetoid movements and dystonia represent frequent sequelae [41].

Cortical and deep venous thrombosis without sinus thrombosis involvement is uncommon and presently difficult to diagnose [42]. The principal symptoms are: headache, focal neurological signs, partial complex or secondary generalized seizures, and consciousness disturbances. Mild intracranial hypertension has been reported in association with headache, nausea and vomiting, but without any signs of papilledema in one fourth of patients. Transient altered consciousness may be linked to seizure generalization, and severe consciousness impairment could be due to an involvement of deep structures [43].

Cavernous sinus thrombosis is rare and represents about 0.5–2% of all cerebral venous thrombosis [5, 44]; it can have infective etiology especially in younger patients, and has characteristic clinical features. Often, the onset in the anterior cavernous sinus thrombosis is abrupt with headache, ocular pain, chemosis, proptosis, ocular nerve palsy (III, IV, VI and the ophthalmic division of V) and fever in the case of infective etiology. In some cases, ocular nerve palsy can be the exclusive symptom. Posterior cavernous sinus thrombosis, spreading to the inferior petrosal sinus, may cause palsies of cranial nerves VI, IX, X and XI without proptosis, and involvement of the superior petrosal sinus may be accompanied by a V nerve palsy [45].

Internal jugular vein can be affected by cerebral venous thrombosis. In most cases, the thrombosis extends from the sigmoid sinus. Swelling and pain in the mastoid region, and a palpable, tender thrombosed vein can be observed. In other cases, thromboses of the internal jugular vein can be the consequence of long-term venous access [46]. Jugular vein thrombosis is most commonly asymptomatic when isolated.

Also the patient's age can determine different patterns of symptoms.

Cerebral venous thrombosis in neonates is considered to be rare and few studies on neonatal cerebral venous thrombosis are available. Cerebral venous thrombosis in neonates can be difficult to diagnose due to its symptoms which often are nonspecific and may lead to cognitive impairment, motor impairment and epilepsy [47]. In a series of 42 neonates, seizures were the most common presentation and occurred in 57% of patients followed by respiratory distress syndrome (19%) and apnea (19%). Poor feeding/weight loss was present in 12%, and acidosis, hypotonia, lethargy and hypertonia were less frequently described. Palpebral ecchymosis and cerebral venous thrombosis were described in a near-term infant [30]. Fifty percent of neonates had involvement of a single sinus, most commonly the sagittal sinus; 50% had simultaneous involvement of multiple sinuses [48].

Cerebral venous thrombosis in newborns, infants and children has a similar clinical picture: lethargy, headache, vomiting, seizures, focal signs are common. In children, thrombosis often affects the superficial venous system. Onset is usually acute in the 83% of cases [49]. Systemic illness (sinusitis, mastoiditis, dehydration) can be present [see the chapter by Yager et al., this vol., pp. 122–131].

When cerebral venous thrombosis affects elderly patients [50], isolated intracranial hypertension syndrome and severe headache are less common, whereas depressed consciousness and mental status changes are more frequent. The prognosis for elderly patients is usually considerably worse. In a series of patients affected by cerebral venous thrombosis, only 49% of elderly patients (≥65 years old) had complete recovery versus 82% in younger patients, whereas 27% died and 22% were dependent at the end of the follow-up versus 7 and 2%, respectively, in younger patients. There were no differences between the two groups in the site and number of occluded sinuses and the presence and type of parenchymal lesions.

References

1 Bousser MG, Ross Russel RW: Cerebral Venous Thrombosis. London: W.B. Saunders, 1997.

2 Bousser MG, Chiras J, Bories J, et al: Cerebral venous thrombosis. A review of 38 cases. Stroke 1985;16:199–213.

3 Hennerici M, Bogousslavsky J, Sacco RL (eds): Clinical Practice Series: Stroke. Elsevier, Philadelphia, 2005.

4 Kuehnen J, Schwartz A, Neff W, Hennerici M: Cranial nerve syndrome in thrombosis of the transverse/sigmoid sinuses. Brain 1998;121:381–388.

5 Bousser MG: Cerebral venous thrombosis: diagnosis and management. J Neurol 2000;247: 252–258.

6 Purvin VA, Trobe JD, Kosmorsky G: Neuro-ophthalmic features of cerebral venous obstruction. Arch Neurol 1995;52:880–886.

7 Biousse V, Ameri A, Bousser MG: Isolated intracranial hypertension as the only sign of cerebral venous thrombosis. Neurology 1999;53:1537.

8 De Bruijn SF, de Haan RJ, Stam J: Clinical features and prognostic factors of cerebral venous sinus thrombosis in a prospective series of 59 patients. For The Cerebral Venous Sinus Thrombosis Study Group. J Neurol Neurosurg Psychiatry 2001;70:105–108.

9 Crassard I, Bousser MG: Cerebral venous thrombosis. J Neuro-Ophthalmol 2004;24:156–163.

10 De Veber G, Andrew M, Adams C, Bjornson B, Booth F, Buckley DJ, Camfield CS, David M, Humphreys P, Langevin P, MacDonald EA, Gillett J, Meaney B, Shevell M, Sinclair DB, Yager J; Canadian Pediatric Ischemic Stroke Study Group: cerebral sinovenous thrombosis in children. N Engl J Med 2001;345:417–423.

11 Masuhr F, Busch M, Amberger N, Ortwein H, Weih M, Neumann K, Einhaupl K, Mehraein S: Risk and predictors of early epileptic seizures in acute cerebral venous and sinus thrombosis. Eur J Neurol 2006;13:852–856.

12 Canhao P, Ferro JM, Lindgren AG, Bousser MG, Stam J, Barinagarrementeria F; ISCVT Investigators: Causes and predictors of death in cerebral venous thrombosis. Stroke 2005;36:1720–1725. Epub 2005 Jul 7.

13 Einhaupl K, Bousser MG, de Bruijn SF, Ferro JM, Martinelli I, Masuhr F, Stam J: EFNS guideline on the treatment of cerebral venous and sinus thrombosis. Eur J Neurol 2006;13:553–559.

14 Ferro JM, Correia M, Rosas MJ, Pinto AN, Neves G; Cerebral Venous Thrombosis Portuguese Collaborative Study Group [Venoport]: Seizures in cerebral vein and dural sinus thrombosis. Cerebrovasc Dis 2003;15:78–83.

15 Manzano Palomo S, Egido Herrero JA, Saiz Ayala A, Jorquera Moya M: Transient ischemic attack: the only presenting syndrome of sinus thrombosis. Neurologia 2006;21:155–158.

16 Straub J, Magistry MR, Delavelle J, Landis T: Facial palsy in cerebral venous thrombosis; transcranial stimulation and pathophysiological considerations. Stroke 2000;31:1766–1769.

17 Garcin R, Pestel M: Thrombophlebites cerebrales. Paris, Masson, 1949.

18 Symonds CP: Hydrocephalus and focal cerebral symptoms in relation to thrombophlebitis of the dural sinuses and cerebral veins. Brain 1937;60:531–550.

19 Bousser MG, Barnett HJM: Cerebral venous thrombosis; in Barnett HJM, Mohr JP, Stein BM, Yatsu FM (eds): Stroke, Pathophysiology, Diagnosis, and Management. New York, Churchill Livingstone, 1998.

20 Oppenheim C, Domigo V, Gauvrit JY, Lamy C, Mackowiak-Cordoliani MA, Pruvo JP, Meder JF: Subarachnoid haemorrhage as the initial presentation of dural sinus thrombosis. AJNR Am J Neuroradiol 2005;26:614–617.

21 Jenkins M, Hussain N, Lee D, Jog MS: Reversible parkinsonism and MRI diffusion abnormalities in cortical venous thrombosis. Neurology 2001;57:364–366.

22 Hart RG, Carter JE: Pseudotumor cerebri and facial pain. Archives of Neurology 1982;39:440–445.

23 Ko YC, Chen WT, Lin PK, Hsu WM, Liu JH: Cerebral venous thrombosis presenting as acute visual loss. Br J Ophthalmol 2001;85:1140–1141.

24 Murray BJ, Llinas R, Caplan LR, Scammell T, Pascual-Leone A: Cerebral deep venous thrombosis presenting as acute micrographia and hypophonia. Neurology 2000;54:751–753.

25 Newman DS, Levine SR, Curris VL, et al: Migraine-like visual phenomena associated with cerebral venous thrombosis. Headache 1989;29:82–85.

26 Crassard I, Biousse V, Bousser MG, et al: Hearing loss revealing lateral sinus thrombosis in a patient with factor V Leiden mutation. Stroke 1997;28:867–870.

27 Ploner CJ, Kupsch A: Ocular flutter in a patient with intracranial hypertension following cerebral venous thrombosis. Neurology 2002;59:959.

28 Fukutame T, Shimoe Y, Hattori T: Dizziness when eating: an unusual isolated presentation of cerebral venous thrombosis. Intern Med 2001;40:961–963.

29 Roy PM, Gras E: Cerebral venous thrombosis. N Engl J Med 2003;349:1730.

30 Fumagalli M, Ramenghi LA, Mosca F: Palpebral ecchymosis and cerebral venous thrombosis in a near term infant. Arch Dis Child Fetal Neonatal Ed 2004;89:530.

31 Solheim O, Skeidsvoll T: Transient global amnesia may be caused by cerebral vein thrombosis. Med Hypotheses 2005;65:1142–1149.

32 Goldberg AL, Rosenbaum AE, Wang H, et al: Computed Tomography of dural sinus thrombosis. J Comput Assist Tomogr 1986;10:16–20.

33 El Ameri A, Bousser MG: Cerebral venous thrombosis. Neurol Clin 1992;10:87–111.

34 Cantu C, Barinagarrementeria F: Cerebral venous thrombosis associated with pregnancy and puerperium. Review of 67 cases. Stroke 1993;24:1880–1884.

35 Jacobs K, Moulin T, Bogousslavsky J, Woimant F, Dehaene I, Tatu L, Besson G, Assouline E, Casselman J: The stroke syndrome of cortical vein thrombosis. Neurology 1996;47:376–382.

36 Dorndorf D, Wessl K, Kessler C, et al: Thrombosis of right vein of Labbe: radiological and clinical findings. Neuroradiology 1993;35:202–204.

37 Jones BV: Case 62: lobar hemorrhage from thrombosis of the vein of Labbe. Radiology 2003;228: 693–696.

38 Thomas B, Krishnamoorthy T, Purkayastha S, Kumar Gupta A: Isolated left vein of Labbe thrombosis. Neurology 2005;65:1135.

39 Walter M, Van den Bergh WM, van der Schaaf I, van Gijn J: The spectrum of presentations of venous infarction caused by deep cerebral vein thrombosis. Neurology 2005;65:192–196.

40 Nakazato Y, Sonoda K, Senda M, Tamura N, Araki N, Tanahashi N, Shimazu K: Case of straight sinus venous thrombosis presenting as depression and disorientation due to bilateral thalamic lesions. Rinsko Shikeigaku 2006;46:652–654.

41 Barnett HJM, Mohr JP, Stein BM, Yatsu FR (eds): Stroke: Pathophysiology, Diagnosis and Management. New York, Churchill Livingston, 1998.
42 Sagduyu A, Sirin H, Mulayim S, Bademkiran F, Yunten N, Kitis O, Calli C, Dalbasti T, Kumral E: Cerebral cortical and deep venous thrombosis without sinus thrombosis: clinical MRI correlates. Acta Neurol Scand 2006;114:254–260.
43 Crawford SC, Digre KB, Palmer CA, Bell DA, Osborn AG: Trhombosis of the deep venous drainage of the brain in adults. Analysis of seven cases with review of the literature. Arch Neurol 1995;52:1101–1108.
44 Milandre L, Guerriot C, Girard L: Les thromboses veineuses cerebrales: etude de l'evolution. Ann Med intern 1988;139:544.
45 Ropper AH, Brown RH: Adams and Victor's: Principles of Neurology, Eighth Edition. McGraw-Hill, New York, 2005.
46 Agnelli G, Verso M: Therapy insight: venous-catheter-related thrombosis in cancer patients. Nat Clin Pract Oncol 2006;3:214–222.
47 Carvalho KS, Bodensteiner JB, Connolly PJ, Garg BP: Cerebral venous thrombosis in children. J Child Neurol 2001;16:574–580.
48 Fitzgerald KC, Williams LS, Garg BP, Carvalho KS, Golomb MR: Cerebral sinovenous thrombosis in the neonate. Arch Neurol 2006;63:405–409.
49 Sebire G, Tabarki B, Saunders DE, Leroy I, Liesner R, Saint-Martin C, Husson B, Williams AN, Wade A, Kirkham FJ: Cerebral venous sinus thrombosis in children: risk factors, presentation, diagnosis and outcome. Brain 2005;128:477–489. Epub 2005 Feb 7.
50 Ferro JM, Canhao P, Bousser MG, Stam J, Barinagarrementeria F; ISCVT Investigators: Cerebral vein and dural sinus thrombosis in elderly patients. Stroke 2005;36:1927–1932. Epub 2005 Aug 11.
51 Ferro JM: Cerebral venous thrombosis. J Neuroradiol 2002;29:231–239.

Dr. Maurizio Paciaroni
Stroke Unit and Division of Cardiovascular Medicine
Department of Internal Medicine, University of Perugia
Santa Maria della Misericordia Hospital
Via Dottori, Sant'Andrea delle Fratte, IT–06126 Perugia (Italy)
Tel./Fax +39 075 5782 765, E-Mail maurizio.paciaroni@med.unipg.it

Caso V, Agnelli G, Paciaroni M (eds): Handbook on Cerebral Venous Thrombosis.
Front Neurol Neurosci. Basel, Karger, 2008, vol 23, pp 89–95

Headache and Cerebral Vein and Sinus Thrombosis

Andrea Alberti, Michele Venti, Sergio Biagini

Stroke Unit and Division of Cardiovascular Medicine, Department of Internal Medicine, University of Perugia, Santa Maria della Misericordia Hospital, Sant' Andrea delle Fratte, Perugia, Italy

Abstract

Headache is the most frequent and often the earliest symptom of cerebral vein and sinus thrombosis (CVT). Intracranial hypertension, vein distension and venous infarction alone or in combination are thought to be the principal mechanisms in the pathophysiology of CVT headache. The absence of specific features and the possibility of presentation without associated neurological signs can make its recognition difficult. The early diagnosis of an association of headache with CVT is crucial for patient well being. Physicians must always consider the possibility of CVT in patients with recent headache, even in the absence of neurological signs or a negative brain CT that seem to rule it out. History of cancer, recent head injury, recurrent venous thrombosis, autoimmune diseases, puerperium and/or pregnancy and the use of oral contraceptives should all raise the attention of the physician for a possible CVT.

Copyright © 2008 S. Karger AG, Basel

Headache with its widely varied etiologies and clinical manifestations is one of the most common symptoms that a physician must evaluate in an emergency room setting. While headache most often has a benign cause, in a small percentage of cases it can be a sign of a serious underlying disease. One of these uncommon but serious causes of headache include cerebral vein and sinus thrombosis (CVT). In fact, headache is the most frequent and earliest symptom of CVT [1]. For this, headache is the principal reason patients with CVT arrive at the emergency room. Since an appropriate treatment influences prognosis, an early recognition of the association of headache with CVT can prove to be lifesaving for the patient.

Table 1. Principal clinical signs of patients with cerebral venous thrombosis

Study	Headache	Papilledema	Seizures	Focal signs	Altered consciousness
Bousser et al. [2] (n = 110)	81	51	42	38	30
Daif et al. [3] (n = 40)	82	80	10	27	10
de Bruijn et al. [4] (n = 59)	95	41	47	46	39
Fink et al. [5] (n = 25)	96	42	40	60	NR
Ferro et al. [6] (n = 624)	89	28	39	52	NR
Agostoni [7] (n = 57)	86	NR	35	52	21
Appenzeler et al. [8] (n = 24)	75	54	NR	54	21
Stolz et al. [9] (n = 79)	73	30	39	57	37

The data are reported in percentages. NR = Not reported.

Table 2. Headache attributed to cerebral venous thrombosis: diagnostic criteria of the International Classification of Headache Disorders [2]

A. Any new headache, with or without neurological signs, fulfilling criteria C and D
B. Neuroimaging evidence of cerebral venous thrombosis
C. Headache (and neurological signs if present) develops in close temporal relation to CVT
D. Headache resolves within 1 month after appropriate treatment

Headache Characteristics

Although cerebral venous thrombosis has a wide spectrum of clinical presentations, thus capable of mimicking numerous other disorders, headache is in all series the predominant symptom. It is present in 75–95% of cases [2–9], as illustrated in table 1. Headache is frequently associated with neurological signs, accompanying the four principal syndromes of CVT: focal sign syndrome, isolated intracranial hypertension, cavernous sinus syndrome, subacute encephalopathy [see the chapter by Paciaroni et al., this vol., pp. 77–88]. The International Headache Society [10] has defined the diagnostic criteria for headache in CVT (table 2). Headache in CVT has no specific characteristics and its clinical presentation could be influenced by several factors: the site and degree of the venous thrombosis, the patient's age and the time between onset and admittance to hospital.

Age

Headache is reported less frequently in the elderly than in the young; this is probably related to a lower frequency of intracranial hypertension in the elderly because of a protective presence of brain atrophy and/or diminished reactivity in pain system [11].

Mode of Onset and Temporal Profile

CVT headache usually has a gradual subacute onset over several days, tending to be persistent, but can also be initially intermittent, worsening over time. With time, CVT headache usually becomes refractory to common analgesics and persisting at night. Headache of this type is often exacerbated by physical activity or other Valsalva maneuvers and worsened with recumbence. CVT headache can sometimes have an abrupt onset developing in less than 24 h [9] and in up to 10% of cases this headache has a thunderclap sudden onset [12–14]. Knowledge of this onset modality is very important because this headache type can be clinically indistinguishable from subarachnoid hemorrhages.

Site

It is diffused but not infrequently reported in the literature as being localized [8].

Intensity

Moderate/severe intensity is prevalent.

Type

It is often aggravating and can be of a throbbing type.

Accompanying Symptoms

Nausea and/or vomiting, phonophobia are the most frequent.

Unusual Presentations

Headache associated with unilateral palatial tinnitus in sigmoid sinus thrombosis [15], headache with cluster headache symptoms [16] or migraine such as those without or with aura [17, 18] have been reported. CVT headache can also develop after diagnostic lumbar puncture, thereby initially mimicking a postural headache [19].

Isolated Headache

Even though headache is the most frequent symptom of CVT, it is usually associated with other neurological signs. A recent study [12] has investigated the characteristics of headache from a prospective study of 123 consecutive patients with CVT, where headache was the only symptom in the absence of intracranial hypertension, meningitis or other intracranial lesions. This study revealed headache as the only manifestation of CVT in 14% (17/123) of patients. The lateral sinus was the most frequently involved sinus (88%) and all but one of the subjects, with isolated unilateral sinus thrombosis had a unilateral headache, ipsilateral to the thrombosis. Here, the most frequently reported characteristics of headache were: progression, persistence and severity both unilateral and throbbing. A few patients had sudden onset and 3 patients presented thunderclap headache. Headache improved within a few days following CVT treatment and prognosis in all cases was good. The authors hypothesized that the pathogenesis of headache, in absence of intracranial hypertension, was due to an irritation of the nerve fibers in the walls of the occluded sinus. Headache can sometimes be the sole neurological sign of CVT; thus, the use of magnetic resonance imaging is justified when in the presence of a patient suffering from a recent headache [20] even when both neurological examination and CT are normal.

Pathophysiology

All of the processes that determine the inflammation, distension, or traction of any of the intracranial algosensitive structures can cause headache. Although headache can sometimes be due to the causes of CVT, such as an infection, it is more often the consequence of venous occlusion.

It can be hypothesized that several mechanisms might be acting alone or in combination [21]. Intracranial hypertension: the obstruction of the large venous sinus, such as the sagittal superior sinus, determines a clinical picture of symptomatic intracranial hypertension. Distension of veins and sinuses: venous sinus occlusion caused by thrombosis determines the distension of pain-sensitive structures of both veins and sinuses. Venous infarction: the obstacle to the blood reflux causes cortical hematic infarcts with subsequent cortical irritation and inflammation.

Management

Headache usually improves rapidly after the administration of heparin. Initially headache can be treated with acetaminophen or when persistent with opioids. It is preferable to avoid the use of Aspirin or other NSAIDs for the concomitant treatment with anticoagulants. Puncture lumbar quickly improves headache due to intracranial hypertension and is particularly indicated when there are disturbances of vision.

Outcome

International diagnostic criteria report that CVT headache resolves within 1 month after an appropriate treatment and is rarely reported as a sequel of CVT [10]. However, in regular clinical practice is it common to visit patients who have developed a new and disabling headache after CVT. In our personal series, 30% (6/20) of CVT patients developed a new chronic headache mostly with tension type characteristics within 6 months, while the patients suffering from migraine before CVT continued to experience migraine attacks. This is an important information because, although the recurrence of CVT is unusual, one problem could be represented by the presentation of a new headache in the follow-up of patients with CVT.

In a 3-year clinical outcome study [22] on consecutive patients with cerebral venous thrombosis, 60% (29/48) of patients developed headache: migraine characteristics (n = 14), tension type headache (n = 13) and others (n = 2). In a further study [9], at a mean follow-up of 44 months, 25% (6/24) of CVT patients developed a new chronic headache with migraine characteristics. All except one of these patients had a parenchyma involvement with superior sagittal sinus thrombosis. In the study by Cumurciuc et al. [12] 30% of patients with CVT had developed a new onset of headache within 3 months in the absence of intracranial hypertension or other intracranial lesions. In the study by Buccino et al. [23], that studied the neurological and cognitive long-term outcome in patients with CVT on 34 patients at 3.5 months follow-up, 29% of patients had suffered from a new recurrent headache following the disease, making the headache the most frequent symptom at outcome for CVT patients; 4 of these patients developed depression. Migraine and tension type headaches are very common in the general population. Many observations have been reported suggesting a close relationship between headache and the regulation of mood [24]. Being so, mood disturbance as a consequence of CVT may play an important role in the pathogenesis of the new headache (see chapter complications of cerebral vein and sinus thrombosis).

Headache: When to Suspect CVT?

Today cerebral vein and sinus thrombosis is widely considered to be underdiagnosed. Headache is the most frequent symptom of CVT but the absence of

Table 3. Warning signals for secondary headache

- First or worst
- Abrupt onset
- Subacute headache with increasing frequency or severity
- Headache brought by exertion or Valsalva maneuver; worse upon recumbence, or orthostatism
- Systemic symptoms and/or signs such fever, vomiting
- Headache associated with neurological symptoms and/or signs

other specific features and the possibility of presentation without associated neurological signs can make its diagnosis difficult. In a study by Ferro et al. [25], the hospital admission of patients with cerebral vein and dural sinus thrombosis was negatively associated with the presence of headache alone. Thus, all headaches require a careful assessment of the patient's history and results from physical examination. The presence of warning signs, reported in table 3, should prompt diagnostic testing for secondary headache [26–29]. History of cancer, recent head injury, recurrent venous thrombosis, autoimmune diseases such as systemic lupus erythematous, puerperium and/or pregnancy [30] and the use of oral contraceptives should all raise the attention of the physician for a possible CVT.

Conclusion

The early diagnosis of an association of headache with CVT is crucial for patient well being. CVT-related headache has no specific characteristics and can be the only symptom. Physicians must always consider the possibility of CVT in patients with recent headache, even in the absence of neurological signs or a negative brain CT that seem to rule it out.

References

1 Bousser MG, Ferro JM: Cerebral venous thrombosis: an update. Lancet Neurol 2007;6:162–170.

2 Ameri A, Bousser MG: Cerebral venous thrombosis. Neurol Clin 1992;10:11–87.

3 Daif A, Awada A, Al-Rajeh S, Abduljabbar M, Rahamn A, Obeid T, Malibary T: Cerebral venous thrombosis in adults. A study of 40 cases from Saudi Arabia. Stroke 1995;26:1193–1195.

4 de Bruijn SF, de Haan FJ, Stam J: Clinical features and prognostic factors of cerebral venous thrombosis in a prospective series of 59 patients. J Neurol Neurosurg Psychiatry 2001;70:105–108.

5 Fink JN, McAuley DL: Cerebral venous sinus thrombosis: a diagnostic challenge. Int Med J 2001;7:384–390.

6 Ferro JM, Canhao P, Stam J, Bousser MG, Barinagaarrementeria F: Prognosis of cerebral vein and dural sinus thrombosis: results of the International Study on Cerebral and Dural Sinus Thrombosis (ISCVT). Stroke 2004;35:664–670.

7 Agostoni E: Headache in cerebral venous thrombosis. Neurol Sci 2004;25(suppl 3):S206–S210.

8 Appenzeler S, Zeller CB, Annichino-Bizzachi JM, Costallat LTL, Deus-Silva L, Voetsch B, Faria AV, Zanardi VA, Damasceno BP, Cendes F: Cerebral venous thrombosis: influence of risk factors and imaging findings on prognosis. Clin Neurol Neurosurg 2005;107:371–378.
9 Stolz E, Rahimi A, Gerriets T, Kraus J, Kaps M: Cerebral venous thrombosis: an all or nothing disease? Prognostic factors and long-term outcome. Clin Neurol Neurosurg 2005;107:99–107.
10 Headache Classification Committee of the International Headache Society: Classification and diagnostic criteria of headache disorders, cranial neuralgias, facial pain. Cephalalgia 2004;24 (suppl 1):1–151.
11 Ferro JM, Canhao P, Stam J, Bousser MG, Barinagaarrementeria F: Cerebral vein and dural sinus thrombosis in elderly patients. Stroke 2005;36:1927–1932.
12 Cumurciuc R, Crassard I, Sarov M, Valade D, Bousser MG: Headaches as the only neurological sign of cerebral venous thrombosis: a series of 17 cases. J Neurol Neurosurg Psychiatry 2005;76:1084–1087.
13 DeBruijn SFTM, Stam J, Kappelle LJ; for CVT study group: Thunderclap headache as first symptom of cerebral venous sinus thrombosis. Lancet 1996;348:1623–1625.
14 Schwedt TJ, Matharu MS, Dodick DW: Thunderclap headache. Lancet Neurol 2006;5:621–631.
15 Sigari F, Blair E, Redleaf M: Headache with unilateral pulsatile tinnitus in women can signal dural sinus thrombosis. Ann Otol Rhino Laryngol 2006;115:686–689.
16 Peterlin BL, Levin M, Cohen JA, Ward TN: Secondary cluster headache: a presentation of cerebral venous thrombosis. Cephalalgia 2006;26:1022–1024.
17 Newman DS, Levine SR, Curtis VL, Welch KM: Migraine-like visual phenomena associated with cerebral venous thrombosis. Headache 1989;29:82–85.
18 Slooter AJC, Ramos LMP, Kappelle LJ: Migraine-like headache as the presenting symptom of cerebral venous sinus thrombosis. J Neurol 2002;249:775–776.
19 Aidi S, Chaunu MP, Biousse V, Bousser MG: Changing patterns of headache pointing to cerebral venous thrombosis after lumbar puncture and intravenous high-dose corticosteroids. Headache 1999;39:559–564.
20 Diener HC: Cerebral venous thrombosis – headache is enough. J Neurol Neurosurg Psychiatry 2005;76:1043.
21 Bousser MG, Good J, Kittner SJ, Silberstein SD: Headache associated with vascular disorders; in Silberstein SD, Lipton RB, Dalessio DJ (eds): Wolff's Headache and Other Head Pain. Oxford, Oxford University Press, 2001, pp 349–352.
22 Breteau G, Mounier-Vehier F, Godefroy O, Gauvrit JY, Mackowiak-Cordoliani MA, Girot M, Bertheloot D, Henon H, Leclerc X, Fourrier F, Pruvo JP, Leys DJ: Cerebral venous thrombosis 3-year clinical outcome in 55 consecutive patients. J Neurol 2003;250:29–35.
23 Buccino G, Scoditti U, Patteri I, Bertolino C, Mancia D: Neurological and cognitive long-term outcome in patients with cerebral venous sinus thrombosis. Acta Neurol Scand 2003;107:330–335.
24 Maizels M, Burchette R: Somatic symptoms in headache patients: the influence of headache, diagnosis, frequency, and comorbidity. Headache 2004;44:983–993.
25 Ferro JM, Lopes MG, Rosas MJ, Fontes J: Delay in hospital admission of patients with cerebral vein and dural sinus thrombosis. Cerebrovasc Dis 2005;19:152–156.
26 Drexler ED: Severe headaches. Postgrad Med 1990;87:164–181.
27 Evans RW: Diagnostic testing for the evaluation for headaches. Neurol Clin 1996;14:1–26.
28 Dodick D: Headaches as a symptom of ominous disease. What are the warning signals? Postgrad Med 1997;101:46–50.
29 Bartleson JD: When and how to investigate the patients with headache. Semin Neurol 2006;26: 163–170.
30 Silberstein SD: Headache in pregnancy. Neurol Clin 2004;22:727–756.

Andrea Alberti, MD
Stroke Unit and Division of Cardiovascular Medicine
Department of Internal Medicine, University of Perugia
Santa Maria della Misericordia Hospital
Via Dottori, Sant' Andrea delle Fratte, IT–06126 Perugia (Italy)
Tel./Fax +39 075 578 2765 E-Mail andrea_alberti@hotmail.com

Caso V, Agnelli G, Paciaroni M (eds): Handbook on Cerebral Venous Thrombosis.
Front Neurol Neurosci. Basel, Karger, 2008, vol 23, pp 96–111

Radiological Diagnosis of Cerebral Venous Thrombosis

Magdy Selim, Louis R. Caplan

Division of Cerebrovascular Diseases, Department of Neurology, Beth Israel Deaconess Medical Center, Harvard Medical School, Boston, Mass., USA

Abstract

Radiological studies are essential to confirm the diagnosis of cerebral venous thrombosis (CVT). Over the last few years, innovations in radiological techniques have significantly improved the diagnosis and altered the management of this condition. Magnetic resonance imaging has become the imaging modality of choice for the diagnosis of suspected CVT, and noninvasive magnetic resonance and computed tomography venography have largely replaced conventional angiography for initial evaluation and follow-up. These techniques have high sensitivity for diagnosing CVT. However, they also have pitfalls that can lead to false-positive and -negative results. Conventional cerebral angiography should be reserved for doubtful cases or when endovascular intervention is advocated.

Copyright © 2008 S. Karger AG, Basel

Early diagnosis and treatment of cerebral venous thrombosis (CVT) is essential to minimize morbidity and improve survival. The condition has a broad spectrum of presentation, and recognizing the presence of CVT on clinical grounds often requires a high degree of suspicion. Radiological studies are crucial to establish the definitive diagnosis [1–3]. In this chapter, we discuss the pathophysiology of CVT as it pertains to radiological findings, and the utility of various imaging modalities to confirm the diagnosis of CVT in suspected cases.

Pathophysiological Mechanisms of CVT

Knowledge of the pathophysiological mechanisms of CVT is essential to understand the radiological findings in patients with CVT. Predisposing factors to CVT affect various elements of Virchow's triad by causing: (1) changes in blood constituents leading to hypercoagulability; (2) changes in blood flow and volume, and (3) changes in the vessel wall. These pathophysiological changes result in venous stasis, secondary venous congestion and thrombosis, and subsequent brain edema, which can be localized or diffuse, and cerebral infarction. The imaging findings in CVT mirror these changes, and can be generally divided into indirect and direct signs of CVT [4]. The indirect signs include: (1) parenchymal abnormalities, namely venous infarcts and brain edema; (2) development of collateral venous network, and (3) mastoid air abnormalities. The direct signs are those of interrupted venous flow or occlusion, and visualization of the actual thrombus.

Imaging of CVT

Computerized axial tomography (CT) is usually the first examination performed in most hospitals when CVT is suspected. However, CT may not reliably diagnose CVT in many suspected cases, especially if contrast is not given. Therefore, the use of multiple imaging modalities to confirm the diagnosis of CVT is not uncommon. The use of CT venography (CTV), and magnetic resonance imaging (MRI) and MR venography (MRV) is being increasingly utilized in major centers. In some patients, conventional angiography, once the gold standard for diagnosis, may be ultimately required to confirm the presence of CVT. For descriptive purposes, we will divide the imaging of CVT into: imaging of the brain parenchyma to assess for indirect signs of CVT, and direct imaging of the sinuses and veins to confirm the presence of CVT.

Imaging of the Brain Parenchyma

Computed Axial Tomography

Plain, noncontrast, CT of the brain shows nonspecific subtle abnormalities in most patients with CVT. CT may be interpreted as 'normal' in 25–40% of patients, later proven to have CVT [4, 5]. This is particularly true in patients with isolated increase in intracranial pressure. The main utility of plain CT in patients with suspected CVT is to rule out other pathologies, such as tumors. Contrast administration is ALMOST ALWAYS required to increase the reliability of CT in diagnosing CVT. However, CT, plain or with contrast, cannot unequivocally confirm the diagnosis of CVT in a large number of patients [4, 5]. Additional imaging modalities, such as MRI/MRV, are often needed. Recent

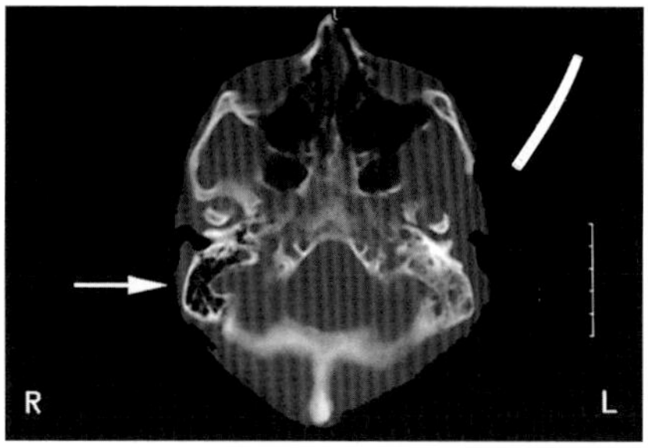

Fig. 1. Plain CT showing erosive changes in the right middle ear and mastoid air cells (arrow) in a patient with right lateral sinus thrombosis.

advances in CTV methodology may decrease the need for additional MRI testing in the future.

The following findings on CT should raise suspicion for CVT in patients whose clinical findings suggest the diagnosis.

Indirect Signs

- Erosion of middle ear structures and changes in the mastoid region (fig. 1). These changes are especially seen in patients with septic lateral sinus thrombosis.
- Hydrocephalus and compression of the fourth ventricle. These changes may be seen in patients with cerebellar sinus thrombosis and venous infarcts.
- Parenchymal changes including venous infarcts (fig. 2a, b), localized or diffuse brain edema and sulcal effacement (fig. 2c), and enhancement of the falx and tentorium. Venous infarcts can be hemorrhagic or nonhemorrhagic. They are present in up to 40% of patients with CVT, the majority of which are hemorrhagic [4, 5]. There are no pathognomonic features to hemorrhagic venous infarcts, and they are often labeled as 'intraparenchymal hemorrhages' upon initial evaluation. However, the following red flags should raise suspicion for venous infarcts: (1) multiplicity; (2) non-arterial territory; (3) subcortical localization; (4) ill-defined appearance, and (5) bilateral involvement of the thalami or basal ganglia [2, 5]. Eccentric hypodensity at the periphery of an intraparenchymal hemorrhage that is present soon after neurological symptom onset suggests that the bleeding developed in an area of brain edema. The edema is caused by CVT-related decreased venous drainage from the edematous portion of the brain. Hypodensity around hypertensive and non-CVT related hemorrhages develops gradually during a 24- to 72-hour period and is usually symmetrical surrounding the hematoma.
- The ventricles are sometimes small and slit-like as a result of increased intracranial pressure and associated edema. Enhancement of the tentorium and/or falx after contrast administration (fig. 3) may signal the presence of dural venous collaterals or venous stasis. Occasionally, isolated gyral or

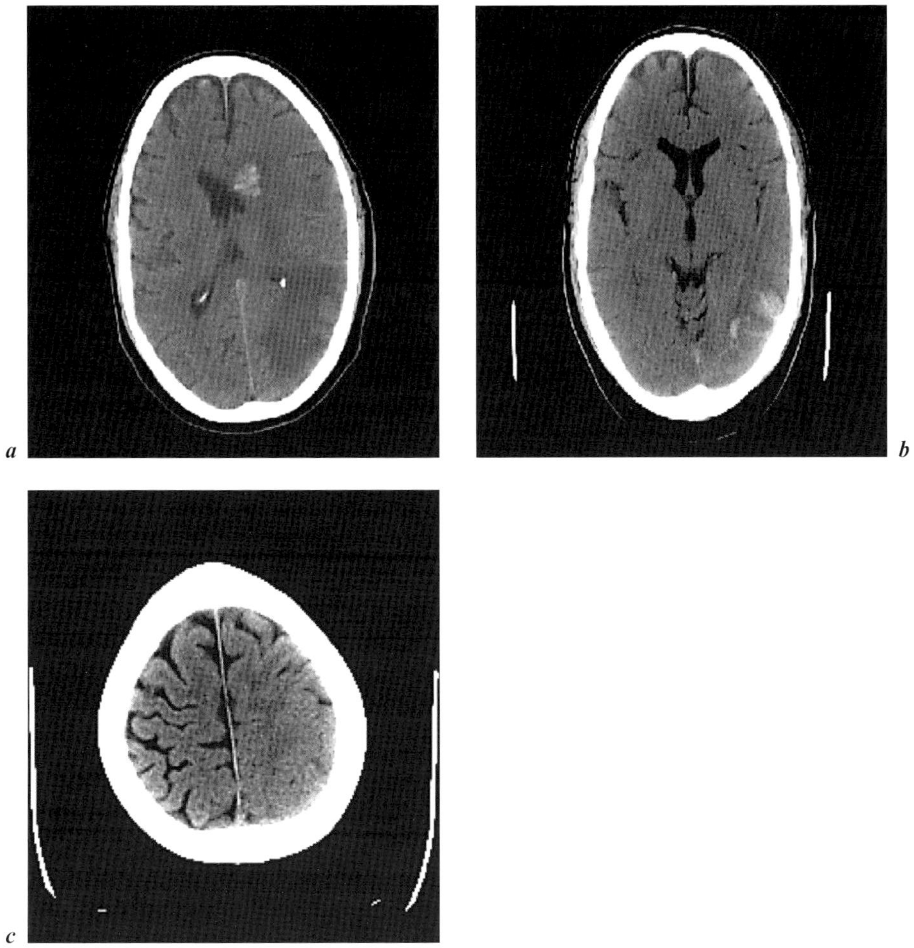

Fig. 2. Plain CT showing left caudate (***a***) and parietal (***b***) hemorrhagic infarcts in a patient with CVT. Note the extent of edema (hypodensity) in the left parieto-occipital region (***a***) and sulcal effacement in the left hemisphere (***c***).

linear enhancement is seen, and may be misinterpreted as 'subarachnoid hemorrhages' (fig. 4).

Direct Signs

- The cord/dense sign. In 2–25% of patients, the fresh thrombus can be visualized as a subtle focus of hyperdensity within the occluded sinus on plain CT (fig. 5). This is best seen within the large straight and superior sagittal sinuses. However, it has poor specificity for CVT since slow flow can produce similar findings [4].

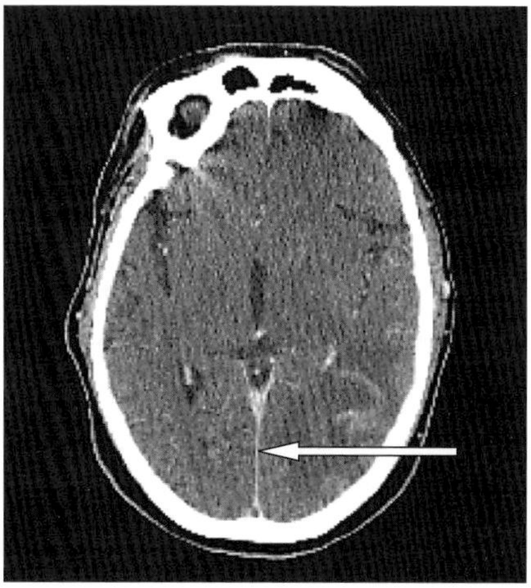

Fig. 3. Contrast-enhanced CT showing enhancement of the falx (arrow).

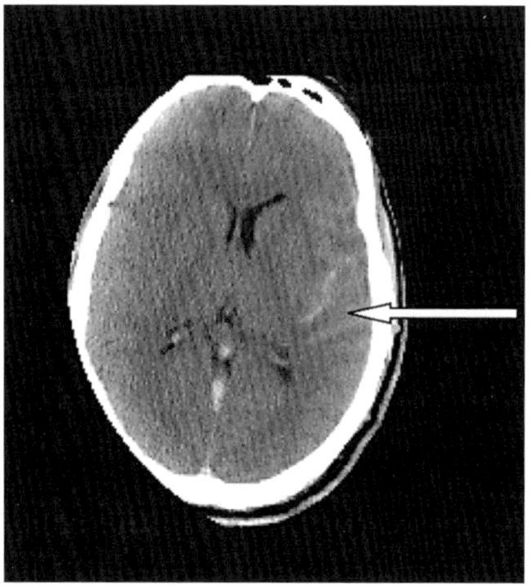

Fig. 4. Plain CT showing an area of linear hyperdensity along the gyri in the left temporal lateral lobe (arrow) in a patient with venous sinus thrombosis. This was initially interpreted as 'subarachnoid hemorrhage'.

- The dense delta (filled triangle) sign. This is seen on plain CT, as a dense triangle (from hyperdense thrombus) within the superior sagittal sinus. It is seen in up to 60% of patients. However, this is not specific and can be observed occasionally in patients with an elevated hematocrit [4].
- The empty delta (empty triangle) sign. This is seen on CT after contrast administration, as a bright triangle surrounding a central hypodense core. It represents contrast enhancement of the dilated collaterals surrounding the clot. It is seen in 25–52% of patients with sagittal, straight, and lateral sinus thrombosis [6]. This sign must be carefully interpreted, since false negatives and false positives are not uncommon [4]. The presence of both

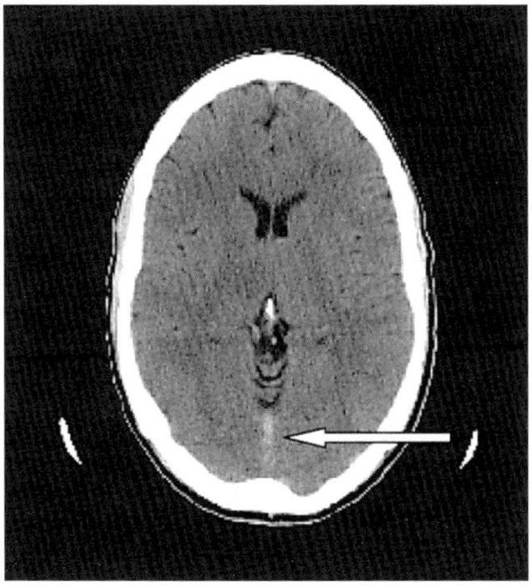

Fig. 5. Plain CT showing the hyperdense fresh thrombus (arrow) in the occluded sinus. This is also referred to as 'the cord' or 'dense sign'. Note the amount of edema (hypodensity) seen in the right thalamic region.

the empty and dense delta signs increases the likelihood of the diagnosis of CVT [4, 5].

Magnetic Resonance Imaging

MRI has become the imaging modality of choice for the diagnosis of suspected CVT. Its multiplanar imaging capabilities and lack of bone artifacts make it more sensitive than CT to parenchymal abnormalities, petechial hemorrhages, thrombus formation, and blood flow. MRI, therefore, is superior to CT in providing definitive evidence for CVT [7, 8]. As seen below, the MRI findings depend on the sequence used and stage (age) of the thrombosis.

Standard Spin Echo T_1- and T_2-Weighted MRI

The main direct sign of CVT on a standard MRI protocol is the lack of expected signal flow void on standard spin echo T_1 and T_2 sequences [7, 8]. Alterations in blood flow and hemoglobin degradation products in thrombosed veins produce signal changes on MR T_1- and T_2-weighted images, which suggest CVT (fig. 6). The appearance and signal intensity of the intraluminal thrombus evolve over time depending on the paramagnetic effects of blood breakdown products, in a manner similar to that of intraparenchymal hemorrhage [4, 7, 8]. Any of the following MRI findings can be seen.

- At a very early acute stage (day 1–5), there is an absence of flow void and the thrombi appear isointense on T_1- and hypointense on T_2-weighted images due to the presence of oxyhemoglobin in the intact red blood cells.

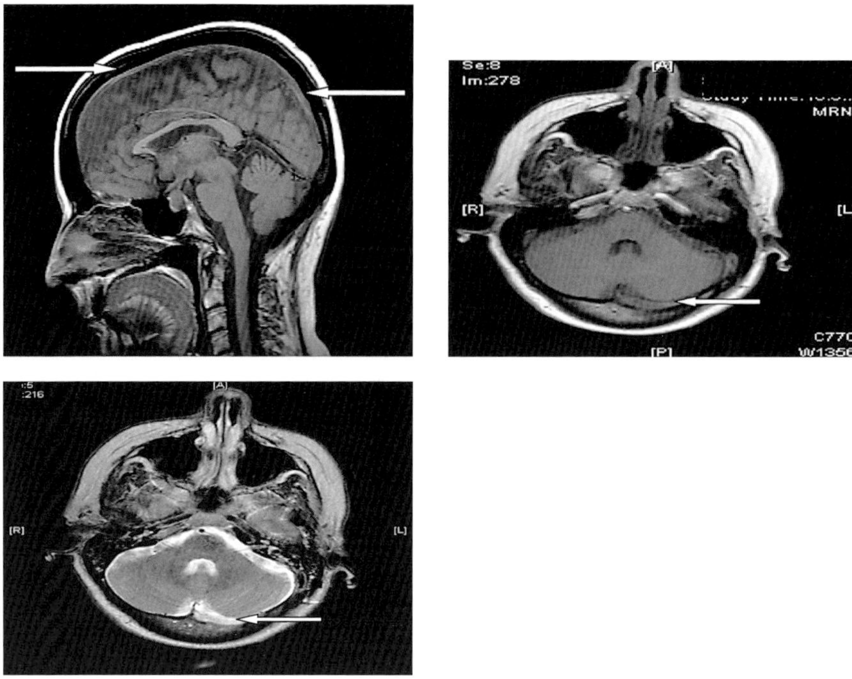

Fig. 6. ***a*** Sagittal T_1-weighted MRI showing a hyperintense signal in a thrombosed superior sagittal sinus (arrows). Axial T_1 (***b***) and T_2 (***c***) MR images show similar signal abnormalities within the thrombosed sinus.

This MRI pattern is rarely seen due to the usual delays in presentation and performing MRI examinations.

- At the subacute stage (day 6–21), the thrombus becomes hyperintense, initially on T_1- (day 6–9) then on T_2-weighted images (day 10–15), due to the conversion of oxyhemoglobin to methemoglobin. Absence of flow void persists. In large sinuses, hyperintensity of the thrombus proceeds from the periphery inwards. This can be seen as a hypointense thrombus surrounded by a circumferential hyperintense rim, 'the target sign'. Increased signal intensity on both T_1 and T_2 images is the most frequent MRI finding in patients with CVT. This pattern lasts until 21–35 days after the onset of thrombosis.
- At the chronic stage (>21–35 days), the MRI pattern is more variable. The thrombosed sinus can either remain totally or partially occluded or can recanalize. In most patients, the chronic thrombus appears heterogenous, becoming progressively isointense on T_1 images and isointense to hyperintense on T_2 images. These findings can last for years and can be mistaken for recurrent CVT.

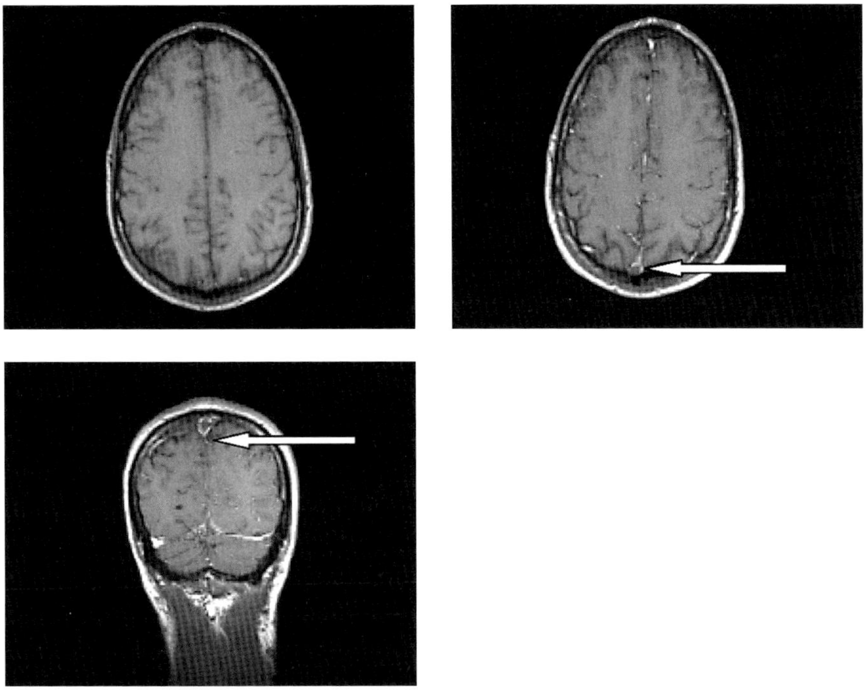

a *b* *c*

Fig. 7. Axial T_1-weighted MRI before (***a***) and after (***b***) gadolinium administration, and coronal sections (***c***). The arrows point to a clot in the sagittal sinus surrounded by enhanced dilated collaterals on postgadolinium images, similar to the empty delta sign described on CT. This is better visualized on coronal sections.

These standard T_1 and T_2 MRI sequences, in isolation, are relatively insensitive since the aforementioned signal changes are variable and often subtle. False negatives and false positives are common, especially in occlusion of small veins, or when there is substantial slowing of blood flow without true occlusion [4, 7]. Furthermore, the lateral sinuses and anterior part of the superior sagittal sinus are often poorly visualized because of the axial-transverse orientation of the imaging sections. Gadolinium administration can increase the sensitivity by showing a delta sign analogous to the one seen on postcontrast CT (fig. 7 and 8). Similarly, the use of coronal sections (fig. 7c and 8b) and variations of repetition time can allow better visualization of the lateral sinuses and differentiating pseudoenhancement due to slow flow from true occlusions.

T2-weighted MRI is sensitive to mucosal changes in the mastoid air sinus. Mastoid abnormalities, ranging from increased T_2 signal, mucosal thickening to accumulation of fluid within the air cells, have been described in 39% of patients with lateral sinus thrombosis [9]. The mastoid abnormalities were

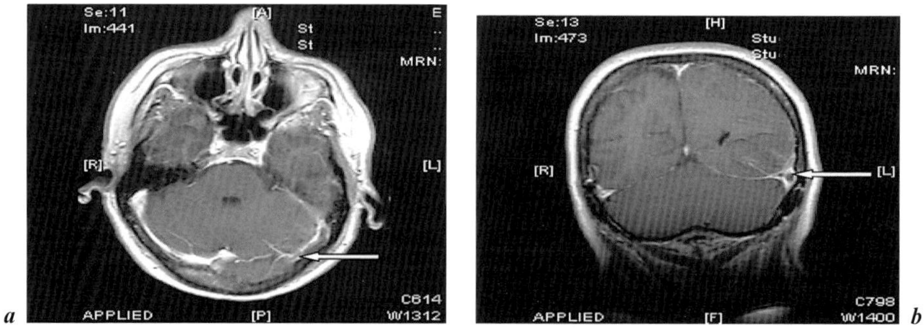

Fig. 8. Gadolinium-enhanced MRI showing decreased flow in the left transverse sinus (***a***), and a corresponding 'empty delta sign' (***b***).

ipsilateral to the thrombosed sinus, and none of these patients had signs of ear disease or mastoiditis. It has been suggested that the mastoid MRI changes in nonseptic lateral sinus thrombosis may be secondary to increased venous pressure in the veins draining the mastoid air cells with subsequent vascular congestion, edema and fluid transudation [9]. This MRI observation may serve as a clue to the presence of an otherwise unrecognized sinus thrombosis.

Echo-Planar T_2 (Susceptibility)-Weighted MRI*

Decreased cerebral venous flow in CVT promotes a local shift in the hemoglobin oxygenation curve toward the formation of deoxyhemoglobin. Deoxyhemoglobin produces a 'magnetic susceptibility effect' and results in signal loss (darkening), which is best seen on T_2*-weighted images. The T_2* MRI sequence can detect the presence of intravenous clot during the acute and subacute phase, seen as an area of hypointensity within the affected sinus (fig. 9) [10, 11]. The T_2* sequence also allows direct visualization of associated venous infarcts that are frequently hemorrhagic, and small petechial hemorrhages (fig. 9). However, the sensitivity and specificity of the T_2* sequence for detecting CVT is unknown.

Diffusion-Weighted MRI

Diffusion-weighted imaging (DWI) abnormalities in patients with CVT are variable and nonspecific (fig. 10). The DWI findings include heterogeneous mixed areas of bright and low signal intensities, multifocal bright lesions similar to those seen in acute arterial strokes, or high signal in clots [12–14]. Hyperintense signal, indicating restricted movement of water molecules, within the thrombosed sinus is seen in 14–41% of patients with CVT (fig. 10c) [15]. However, this is neither sensitive nor complimentary to standard T_1, T_2, and FLAIR images for diagnosing CVT. It has been suggested that the presence of hyperintense signals on DWI in

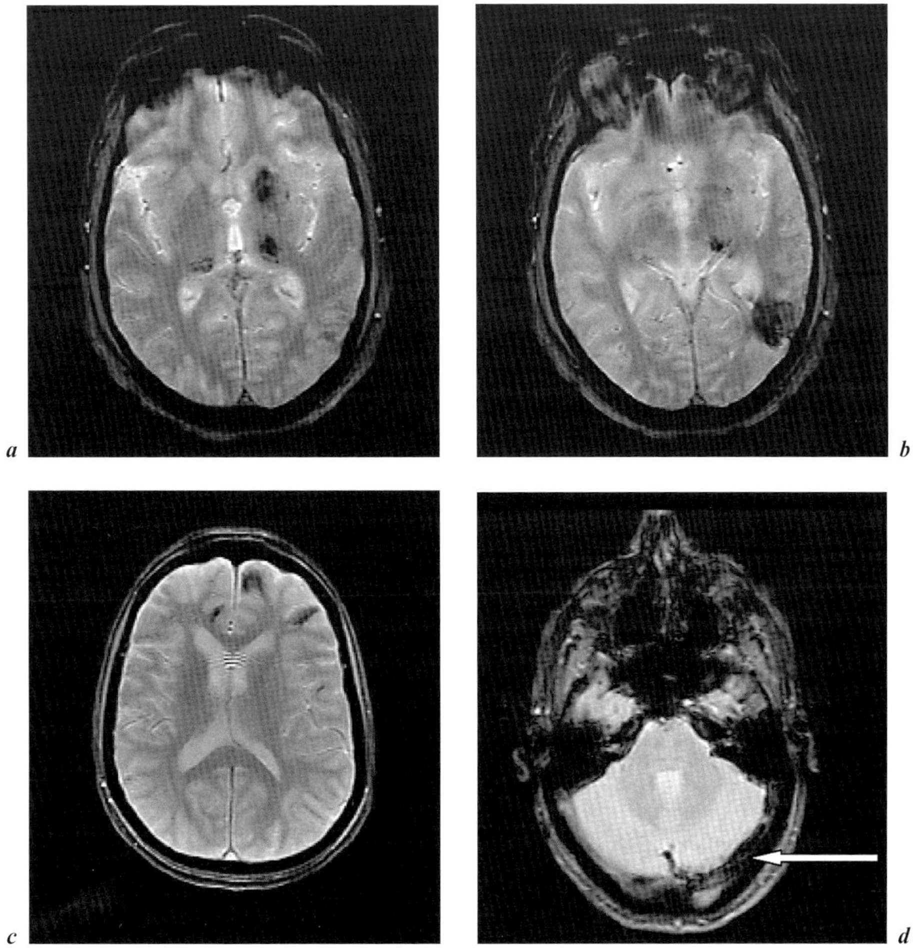

Fig. 9. Echo-planar T_2*-weighted MRI showing multiple susceptibility abnormalities consistent with hemorrhagic infarct (***a–c***), and thrombosed left transverse sinus (***d***). Note the multiple, nonarterial, and bilateral locations of the hemorrhagic lesions. This could be the only clue to an underlying CVT.

occluded veins at the time of diagnosis might be predictive of a low rate of recanalization 2–3 months later [15]. Quantitative assessment of apparent diffusion coefficients of the DWI lesions may be helpful in differentiating between vasogenic and cytotoxic edema, and assessing tissue viability [12, 13]. The main advantage of DWI, thus, lies in its ability to detect subtle abnormalities or subclinical venous congestion and brain swelling before visible parenchymal lesions appear on standard T_1, T_2 and FLAIR MR images [14].

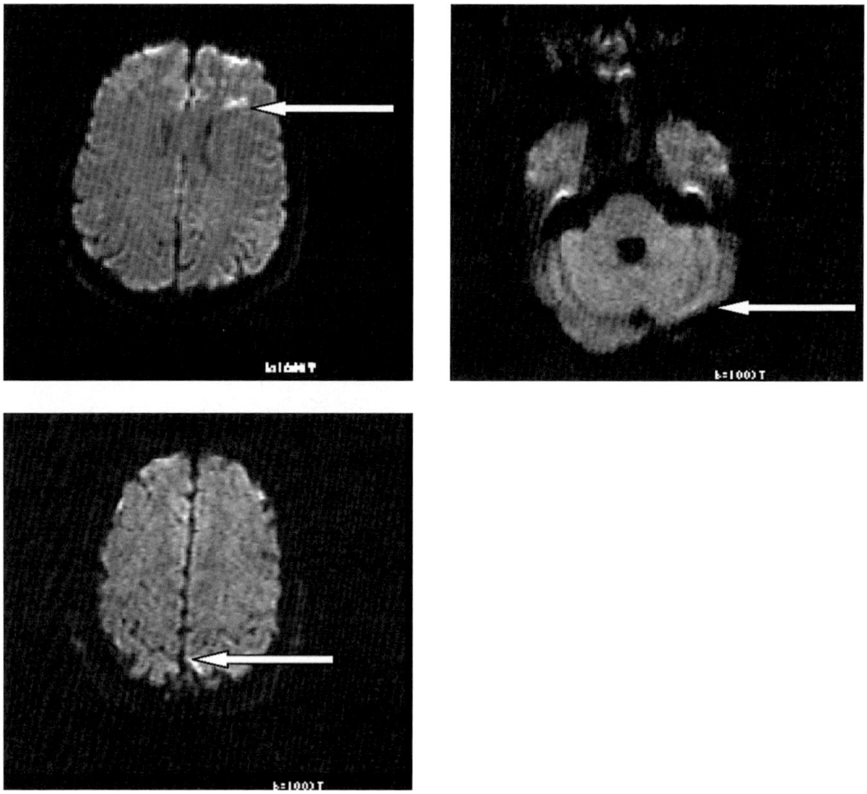

Fig. 10. Diffusion-weighted MRI in a patient with CVT. ***a*** Early infarct. ***b, c*** Intrasinus clot (arrows). ***c*** Hyperintense signal within the thrombosed sinus.

Imaging of the Sinuses and Veins

Direct visualization of the thrombosed sinus is required to conclusively confirm the diagnosis of CVT, regardless of the modality used to image the brain parenchyma. The major cerebral sinuses and veins can be reliably imaged by several techniques, including MRV, CTV, and conventional angiography.

Magnetic Resonance Venography

MRV has become the imaging modality most widely used to establish the diagnosis of CVT. MRV can be performed with time of flight (TOF) or phase contrast techniques (PCT) [7, 16]. TOF relies mainly on flow-related enhancement for producing vascular images, whereas PCT uses velocity-induced phase

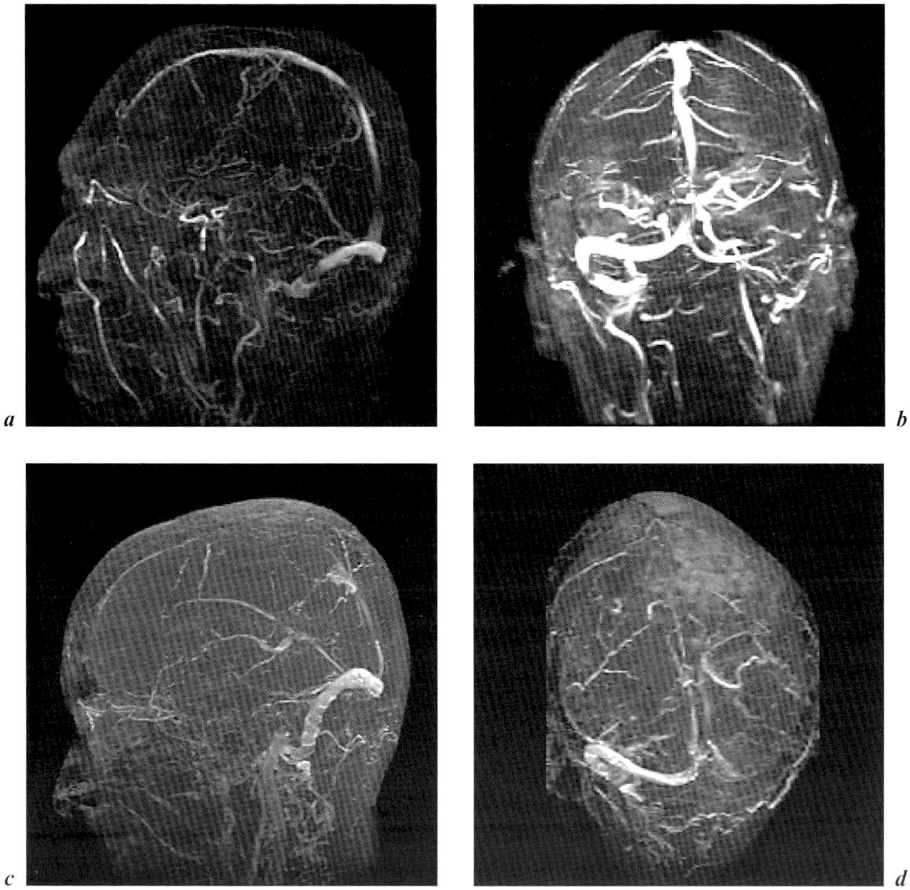

Fig. 11. Magnetic resonance venogram (without gadolinium) in a normal subject (***a, b***) and in a patient with CVT (***c, d***). Note the artifactual flow gaps seen in the superior sagittal sinus and hypoplastic left transverse sinus in ***a*** and ***b***.

shifts to distinguish moving blood flow from the surrounding stationary tissue. Most hospitals utilize TOF technique because of its shorter acquisition time and larger covering volume. Absence of flow signal within a sinus and its nonopacification suggest intraluminal thrombosis (fig. 11). The occluding thrombus often appears hyperintense. This may be difficult to distinguish from the hyperintensity of the flowing blood with TOF, but not PCT. MRV has other limitations that should be emphasized to avoid misleading false-negative or -positive diagnoses [4, 7, 16]. For example, artifactual flow gaps in the nondominant (hypoplastic) transverse sinuses can be seen in up to 30% of normal individuals when using TOF MRV, leading to an erroneous diagnosis of sinus thrombosis (fig. 11a, b) [16].

These are attributed to slow intrasinus blood flow, in-plane flow, or complex blood flow patterns which can result in intrasinus signal loss mimicking occlusion. Also, the saturation of blood flow when the images are parallel to a sinus, particularly the anterior portion of the superior sagittal sinus, can result in loss of signal intensity and false diagnosis of sinus occlusion [7, 16].

These pitfalls are uncommon and can be avoided by setting the slice thickness as small as possible, slice acquisition in the coronal plane to provide maximum coverage of the predominantly anteroposterior direction of dural sinus flow, lowering T_1 of blood through the use of gadolinium [17], and combining the aforementioned findings on standard T_1, T_2 and T_2* sequences with those from MRV [16]. The utility of MRV extends well beyond mere diagnosis of CVT. It is an important, noninvasive, tool to assess for recanalization as a measure of response to anticoagulation therapy.

Cerebral CT Venography

Recently, dynamic spiral CT techniques have been utilized to study the cerebral venous circulation. Spiral cerebral CT venography can be easily and rapidly performed in the acute setting, immediately following noncontrast CT. Filling defects within the affected sinuses, sinus wall enhancement and abnormal venous collaterals are the usual findings (fig. 12). This modality can be particularly useful in hospitals where timely access and availability of MRI or conventional angiography is limited. CTV images are not impaired by in-plane flow signal loss seen with MRV, and may be superior to MRV in visualizing sinuses or smaller veins with low flow [18].

Conventional Angiography

A four-vessel cerebral angiogram allows visualization of the entire venous phase. However, its utility in recent years has declined because of its invasive nature and increased availability of MRI/MRV and CT/CTV techniques. Anteroposterior and lateral films are required. Oblique films are usually needed in patients with suspected sagittal sinus thrombosis, and neck films to see if the jugular vein is occluded. Failure of a sinus/vein to fill (opacify) throughout all or most of its course suggests thrombosis. Dilated, tortuous venous collaterals extending away from the occluded sinus or vein, and a prolonged contrast blush in the brain parenchyma further support the diagnosis (fig. 13). An empty delta sign may also be seen on frontal views in cases of superior sagittal sinus thrombosis. The use of cerebral angiography to diagnose CVT has limitations.

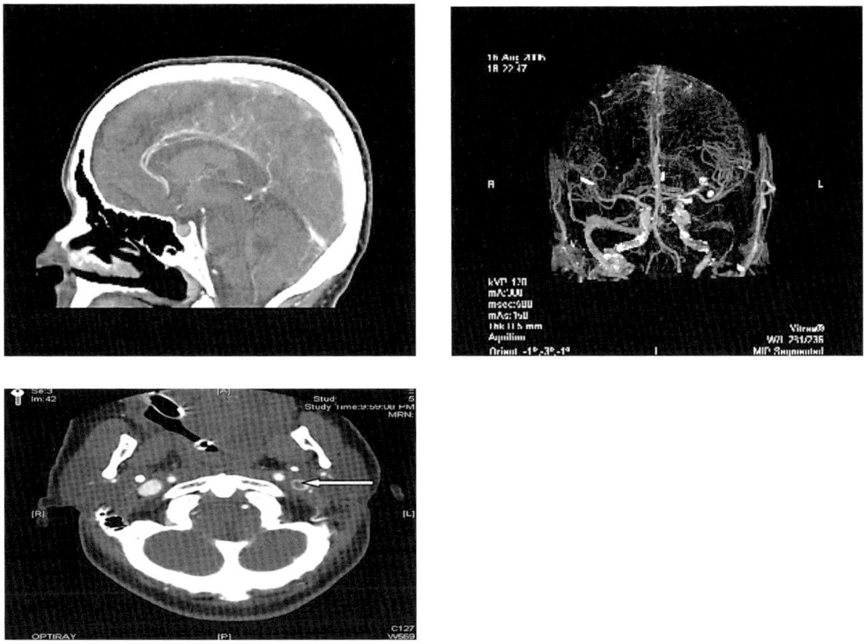

a b c

Fig. 12. ***a*** CT venography showing thrombosed superior sagittal sinus. ***b*** 3-D CTV showing thrombosed left transverse sinus. ***c*** CTA shows thrombosed left internal jugular vein.

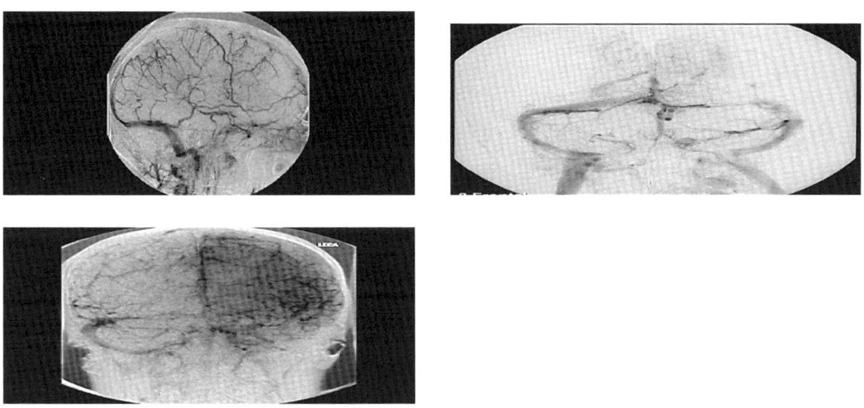

a b c

Fig. 13. Conventional angiography showing thrombosis of the superior sagittal (***a***) and left transverse (***b***) sinuses, and prolonged contrast blush (***c***).

Hypoplastic sinus(es) may not opacify, leading to a false diagnosis of pseudo-occlusion. MRI, together with MRV, is more reliable in differentiating hypoplastic from occluded sinuses as mentioned above. Thrombosis of the cavernous sinus cannot be reliably diagnosed with conventional angiography. The use of conventional angiography is currently limited to patients in whom MRI/MRV is inconclusive, especially those with isolated cortical vein thrombosis, and in cases where intrasinus administration of thrombolytic therapy or interventional recanalization procedures are contemplated.

Transcranial Doppler

Ultrasound techniques may have a role in diagnosing CVT [19] [see also the chapter by Stolz, this vol., pp. 112–121]. Thrombosis of the superior sagittal sinus or deep basal veins of Galen, Labbé or Rosenthal can be associated with increased flow velocities in the deep venous system. It has been suggested that serial transcranial Doppler (TCD) evaluations may be useful in monitoring changes in venous flow and response to treatment. However, available data about the utility of TCD in CVT are limited, and the reliability of TCD findings needs confirmation.

Conclusions

Progress in neuroimaging techniques has made the diagnosis of CVT easier. At present, MRI, combined with MRV, is largely reliable as the sole imaging modality for diagnosing CVT. It is noninvasive, and can show anatomical details of the disturbed venous circulation and secondary parenchymal changes. However, this technique has its pitfalls that can lead to false-positive and -negative results. Conventional cerebral angiography should be reserved for doubtful cases. The use of CTV is rapidly evolving, and is likely to play a larger role in diagnosing CVT in the future.

References

1 Biousse V, Bousser MG: Cerebral venous thrombosis. Neurologist 1999;5:326–349.
2 Stam J: Thrombosis of the cerebral veins and sinuses. N Engl J Med 2005;352:1791–1798.
3 Bousser MG: Cerebral venous thrombosis. Stroke 1999;30:481–483.
4 Provenzale JM, Joseph GJ, Barboriak DP: Dural sinus thrombosis: findings on CT and MR imaging and diagnostic pitfalls. AJR 1998;170:777–783.
5 Rao KCVG, Knipp HC, Wajner EJ: CT findings in cerebral sinus and venous thrombosis. Radiology 1981;140:391–398.
6 Virapongse C, Cazenave C, Quisling R, Sarwar M, Hunter S: The empty delta sign. Radiology 1987;162:779–785.

7 Bianchi D, Maeder PH, Bogousslavsky J, Schnyder P, Meuli RA: Diagnosis of cerebral venous thrombosis with routine magnetic resonance: an update. Eur Neurol 1998;40:179–190.
8 Connor SE, Jarosz JM: Magnetic resonance imaging of cerebral venous sinus thrombosis. Clin Radiol 2002;57:449–461.
9 Fink JN, McAuley DL: Mastoid air sinus abnormalities associated with lateral venous sinus thrombosis. Cause or consequence? Stroke 2002;33:290–292.
10 Selim M, Fink J, Linfante I, Kumar S, Schlaug G, Caplan LR: Diagnosis of cerebral venous thrombosis with echo-planar T_2*-weighted magnetic resonance imaging. Arch Neurol 2002;59: 1021–1026.
11 Idbaih A, Boukobza M, Crassard I, Porcher R, Bousser MG, Chabriat H: MRI of clot in cerebral venous thrombosis: high diagnostic value of susceptibility-weighted images. Stroke 2006;37: 991–995.
12 Chu K, Kang DW, Yoon BW, Roh JK: Diffusion-weighted magnetic resonance in cerebral venous thrombosis. Arch Neurol 2001;58:1569–1576.
13 Wasay M, Bakshi R, Bobustuc G, Dubey N, Cheema Z, Dai A: Diffusion-weighted magnetic resonance imaging in superior sagittal sinus thrombosis. J Neuroimaging 2002;12:267–269.
14 Lovblad KO, Bassetti C, Schneider J, Guzman R, El-Koussy M, Remonda L, Schroth G: Diffusion-weighted MR in cerebral venous thrombosis. Cerebrovasc Dis 2001;11:169–176.
15 Favrole P, Guichard JP, Crassard I, Bousser MG, Chabriat H: Diffusion-weighted imaging of intravascular clots in cerebral venous thrombosis. Stroke 2004;35:99–103.
16 Ayanzen RH, Bird CR, Keller PJ, McCully FJ, Theobald MR, Heiserman JE: Cerebral MR venography: normal anatomy and potential diagnostic pitfalls. AJNR 2000;21:74–78.
17 Liang L, Korogi Y, Sugahara T, Onomichi M, Shigematsu Y, Yang D, Kitajima M, Hiai Y, Takahashi M: Evaluation of the intracranial dural sinuses with a 3D contrast-enhanced MP-RAGE sequence: prospective comparison with 2D-TOF MR venography and digital subtraction angiography. AJNR 2001;22:481–492.
18 Casey SO, Alberico RA, Patel M: Cerebral CT venography. Radiology 1996;198:163–170.
19 Canhao P, Batista P, Ferro JM: Venous transcranial Doppler in acute dural sinus thrombosis. J Neurol 1998;245:276–279.

Magdy Selim, MD, PhD
Assistant Professor of Neurology
Harvard Medical School, Beth Israel Deaconess Medical Center
Department of Neurology, Division of Cerebrovascular Diseases
330 Brookline Avenue, Boston, MA 02215 (USA)
Tel. +1 617 632 8911, Fax +1 617 632 8920, E-Mail mselim@bidmc.harvard.edu

Caso V, Agnelli G, Paciaroni M (eds): Handbook on Cerebral Venous Thrombosis.
Front Neurol Neurosci. Basel, Karger, 2008, vol 23, pp 112–121

Role of Ultrasound in Diagnosis and Management of Cerebral Vein and Sinus Thrombosis

Erwin P. Stolz

Department of Neurology, Justus Liebig University, Giessen, Germany

Abstract

Ultrasound examination of cerebral veins and sinuses is a new application which has been developed in the recent years. In the acute phase of cerebral vein and sinus thrombosis, occlusion of dural sinuses may be diagnosed by transcranial color-coded duplex sonography (TCCS) after echo contrast agent application demonstrating a filling defect. Collateral venous flow can be assessed by both transcranial Doppler sonography and TCCS. However, ultrasonographic techniques are not sensitive enough to exclude cerebral venous thrombosis, but they may complement other imaging techniques. In the follow-up, sonographic findings are related to the functional outcome.

Copyright © 2008 S. Karger AG, Basel

The most frequent symptoms and signs of cerebral venous thrombosis (CVT) are unspecific and include headaches (80–90%), hemiparesis (40–50%), seizures (30–40%), and mental state disorders (20–30%) [1, 2]. In a cohort of emergency room patients presenting with such symptoms, a frequency of CVT of approximately 10% has been found [3], which is far higher than previously thought. Oligosymptomatic cases further complicate diagnostic decisions. This raises the question of suitable screening techniques which can be applied in an emergency department. Venous ultrasound techniques have been developed in the mid-1990s in the hope to be used as a noninvasive, easy to use and cost-effective screening method for CVT.

Examination Technique

Venous anatomy relevant to ultrasound application and the examination technique have been reviewed in detail in another volume of this series [4]. One important anatomic characteristics of the intracranial venous system with relevance for ultrasound examinations is the lack of valves. This implies that the flow direction in cerebral veins and dural sinuses is governed solely by the current pressure gradient.

Only the veins and sinuses located in proximity of the cranial base and the posterior fossa sinuses can be examined by ultrasound techniques. The most important limitation of the technique is the inability to visualize cortical veins and the superior sagittal sinus (SSS) in its frontal, mid-, and posterior part, except for the portion adjacent the confluens sinuum.

In principle, examination can be performed with both conventional transcranial Doppler sonography (TCD) and transcranial color-coded duplex sonography (TCCS) [5]. TCD uses the segments of the circle of Willis as landmarks to identify venous vessels and is thereby limited in the extent of the examination. The clear advantage of TCCS over TCD is that it represents a true imaging method with depiction of parenchymal structures simultaneous with the blood flow information, enabling examination independent of arterial landmarks.

Transcranial Doppler Sonography

Examination usually starts by insonation through the temporal acoustic bone window. The main segments of the circle of Willis serve as landmarks. The deep middle cerebral vein (dMCV) is found in close proximity of the middle cerebral artery mainstem; the postpeduncular part of the basal vein (BV) is best insonated slightly superior of the P2-segment of the posterior cerebral artery [6]. The leading structure towards the cavernous sinus inflow region (sphenoparietal sinus, SPaS, and superior petrosal sinus, SPS) is the carotid siphon; however, a clear anatomic identification of the flow signal is not possible [7]. Flow in these venous vessels is normally directed away from the transducer. The ophthalmic window can be used to examine the superior ophthalmic vein and the cavernous sinus region [7]. Through the occipital foramen, the inferior petrosal sinus (IPS) can be reached in a depth of 9–10 cm using the basilar artery as a leading structure [8]. The venous signal found lateral of the artery displays a flow towards the probe. The occipital bone window provides access to the straight sinus (SRS) with flow directed towards the transducer [9]. However, this ultrasound window is hampered by a high rate of insufficient acoustic penetration [10].

Due to the low venous flow velocities, the pulse repetition frequency generally needs to be reduced and a small sample volume has to be used to prevent masking of the venous signal by the arterial Doppler spectrum. Sometimes it may be necessary to ascertain the venous origin of a Doppler signal by the prompt reactivity upon a brief Valsalva maneuver.

In principle, TCCS uses the same acoustic bone windows as TCD. In order to examine intracranial veins and sinuses, a low-flow sensitive color program with a low wall filter setting has to be used and the pulse repetition frequency needs to be reduced. The color gain is increased to the artifact threshold. Insonation starts in the mesencephalic examination plane with the mesencephalon as the major landmark in B mode. The dMCV is found adjacent to the middle cerebral artery and is best insonated in the transition of the M1 to the M2 segments. The cavernous sinus inflow region is imaged by downward tilt of the transducer to the cranial base. Landmark structure for insonation of the SPaS is the echogenic lesser wing, and for the SPS the echogenic pyramid of the sphenoid bone. Using the mesencephalon as reference plane, for depiction of the BV the transducer is angulated upwards towards the diencephalic plane. The BV is found slightly cranial to the P2 segment of the posterior cerebral artery. All aforementioned structures display a flow away from the probe. Then the B mode depth is increased, so that the contralateral skull becomes visible. Prominent midline structures of the diencephalic insonation plane comprise the echogenic double reflex of the third ventricle and the echogenic pineal gland. The great cerebral vein (of Galen; GCV) is found immediately behind the pineal gland with a flow away from the transducer. In this examination plane, the rostral part of the SSS may be visible. In order to examine the SRS, the anterior tip of the transducer needs to be rotated upwards to align the insonation plane with the plane of the apex of the cerebellar tentorium. The course of the SRS is directed away from the transducer towards the confluens sinuum. Proceeding from this transducer position, the probe is angulated downwards again to depict the contralateral transverse sinus (TS). For examination of the IPS, the same approach is used as for TCD. The medial frontal bone window, which is located paramedially on the forehead, allows the examination of the internal cerebral veins (ICV) [11]. The occipital bone window, located about two finger widths above and paramedially to the external occipital protuberance, allows access to the SRS sinus, the GCV, and the ICV [12].

Normal Values and Reproducibility

Normal values for venous flow velocities are summarized in table 1. No significant differences have been observed between values obtained by TCD or TCCS. In healthy controls, the detection rates of the deep cerebral veins (dMCV, BV, GCV) is high, especially when TCCS is used; however, variable insonation rates have been reported for the posterior fossa sinuses [5]. The

Table 1. Normal values of flow velocities in cerebral veins and sinuses

	Flow velocities	Detection rates, %
TCCS, temporal bone window (n = 250)		
dMCV	4–15/3–11	53–95
BV	7–20/5–15	85–100
GCV	6–32/4–25	84–94
SRS	6–39/4–27	23–82
TS	6–56/5–38	20–84
SSS	6–20/3–14	38–67
TCCS, temporal bone window (n = 43)		
SPaS + SPS	27 ± 17	84
TCCS, occipital (n = 120) and frontal bone windows (n = 75)		
GCV	12–34/7–26	20–34
SRS	7–64/2–43	50–81
ICV	7–22/4–16	13–60
TCD transforaminal bone window (n = 80)		
IPS	20 ± 9	78

Flow velocities are given as range of systolic/diastolic values if not otherwise indicated. DR = Detection rates. Data are based on references [7, 11, 23–26].

reproducibility and interobserver reliability of venous measurements are comparable to those in the arterial system [13]. However, as with all ultrasonographic methods, accuracy is operator-dependent.

Application of Ultrasound in CVT

Ultrasound in the Acute Phase of Illness

First reports on the use of TCD in CVT date back to the 1990s, when high venous flow velocities were found in patients more or less incidentally [14, 15]. These flow signals were interpreted as a consequence of collateral venous flow and were the motivation for systematic studies.

However, even in studies where examiners were not blinded to diagnosis, the rate of pathological examinations ranges from 50 to 100% (table 2), so that CVT cannot be excluded with ultrasonographic methods. Only two studies,

Table 2. Systematic studies of venous transcranial ultrasound in acute CVT

	Reference					
	16	27	28	17	18	21
Method	ce-TCCS	TCD	TCD	3D-TCCS	TCCS	TCCS
Patients with CVT/cohort	8/14	6/6	18/18	3/28	8/8	26/26
Pathological US, %	88	50	100	100	63	69
Pathological findings in deep cerebral veins, %	n.e.	67	17	n. e.	62	56
Pathological findings in sinuses, %	100	33	83	100	38	44
Annotation	only examination of TS	–	–	only examination of TS	–	–
Sensitivity, %	73	–	–	100	–	–
Specificity, %	80	–	–	65	–	–
PPW, %	67	–	–	15	–	–
NPW, %	84	–	–	100	–	–
Reference	MRT/MRA	MRI/MRA DSA	MRI/MRA DSA	MRI/MRA CTA DSA	MRI/MRA DSA	MRI/MRA CTA DSA

US = Ultrasound; ce-TCCS = contrast-enhanced TCCS; 3D-TCCS = three-dimensionally reconstructed TCCS; n.e. = not examined; PPV = positive predictive value; NPV = negative predictive value; DSA = digital subtraction angiography.

both limited to the examination of the TS and using echo-contrast agents, provide data on sensitivity and specificity [16, 17]. In these studies, sensitivity ranges between 73 to 100% and specificity between 65 to 80%. Current data suggest the following diagnostic criteria:

Direct Criteria

Direct criteria comprise the lack of color signal within a dural sinus after application of echo contrast agents. However, thrombotic occlusion or partial thrombosis cannot be differentiated from aplasia or hypoplasia by ultrasound alone. Even three-dimensional reconstruction does not improve the rate of false-positive results [17].

Indirect Criteria

Indirect criteria are based on the detection of venous collateral flow. The following patterns can be observed [5]:

- Due to high venous flow velocities in collaterals, numerous prominent veins are visible even when an arterial presetting of the ultrasound system is used.
- Venous flow velocities are pathologically increased (defined as > mean + 2 standard deviations) as a result of a collateral venous outflow. The extent of the increase in flow velocities depends on the anatomical location, the ability of venous wall distension, the original caliber of the collateral, and the volume flow in relation to the total collateral volume flow. False-positive results may arise when flow velocities in the SPaS and the SPS are measured in proximity of the cavernous sinus, because of the gradual tapering of the diameter, so that measurements should be performed more distally from the cavernous entrance.
- A retrograde flow direction in the BVs is typically found in SRS occlusion. In the proximal part of the TS, flow reversal can be observed when the sinus is distally occluded. The SPS may show a reversed flow when the pressure gradient is directed towards the TS.
- Significant side differences (>50%) for the dMCV and the BV were not observed in normals [18]. Due to the considerable rate of hypoplasias or caliber differences, side differences of flow velocities in paired sinuses have only a diagnostic relevance when venous flow velocities are pathologically increased.

Despite the limitations of the method, transcranial ultrasound provides information on venous hemodynamics, which is not offered by computed tomography angiography (CTA) and conventional time of flight magnetic resonance angiography (MRA), and is therefore complementary to these methods.

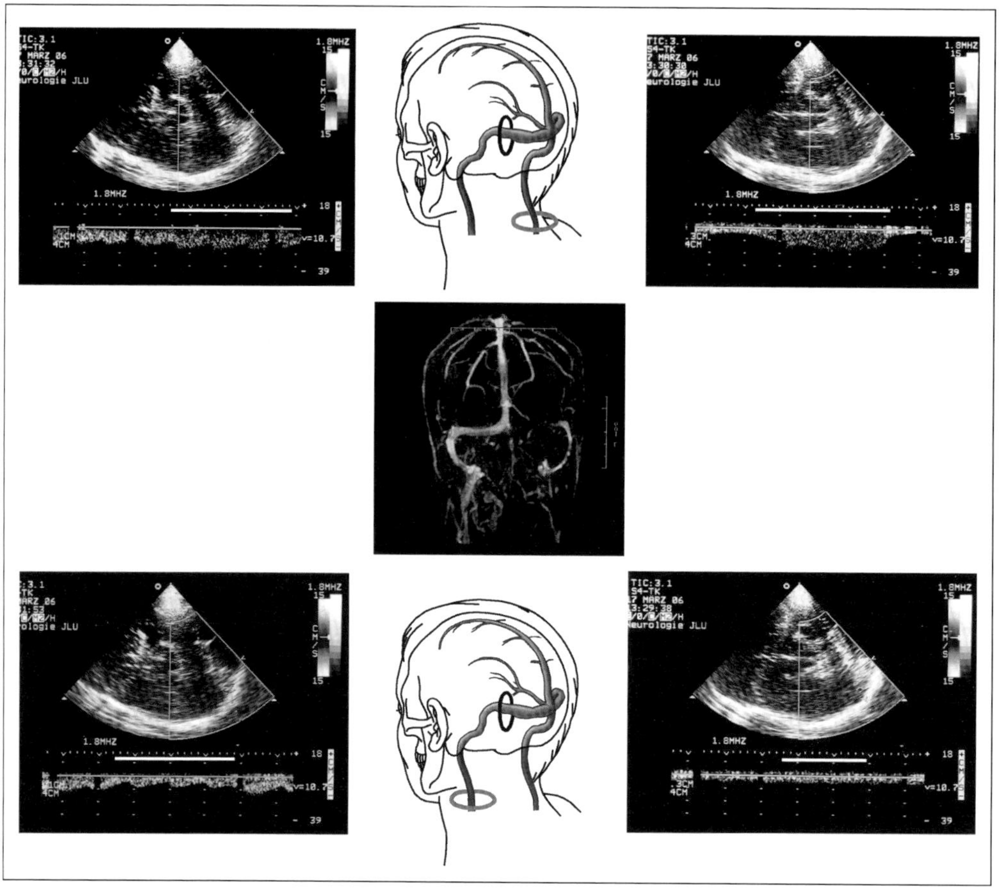

Fig. 1. Functional venous examination. The MRA shows a lack of flow signal in the left TS. Differential diagnoses can either be sinus occlusion, aplasia, or artifact with insufficient sensitivity to detect flow in severe hypoplasia. Upper panel depicts insonation of the TS (dark circle) and short compression of the contralateral jugular vein (gray circle). In the dominant TS, compression (white line) leads to a modest flow velocity increase, in the nondominant TS to a large increase. Lower panel depicts insonation of the TS (dark circle) and compression of the ipsilateral jugular vein (gray circle). Compression (white line) leads to a significant decrease in flow velocities in the dominant TS, while it has little to no effect on the nondominant TS. Compression maneuver could exclude occlusion or aplasia in this case; however, hypoplasia or partial thrombosis cannot be excluded.

Functional Venous Examinations

So far, functional venous ultrasound examinations have been reported for the extracranial venous system: in the supine position, the internal jugular veins are the major drainage pathway, while in the upright position the jugular veins collapse, and the vertebral venous plexus serves as the main outflow tract [19, 20].

Functional venous examinations may also be helpful in clarifying MRA findings relevant to the differential diagnosis of CVT. A frequent, yet not always pathologic finding on MRA is a missing flow signal particularly in the TS. According to our own experience [unpubl. data], insonation of the TS by TCCS and a short compression of the jugular vein may clarify the question whether the TS is patent or occluded (fig. 1). Of course, this approach cannot differentiate between hypoplasia and partial thrombosis.

Ultrasound in the Follow-Up of CVT

Venous transcranial Doppler and duplex sonography are particularly suitable for follow-up examinations. In our own prospective study of 26 patients with acute CVT, an initially normal venous ultrasound examination or normalization within 90 days were significantly associated with an excellent outcome (modified Rankin Scale score 0 or 1) [21]. In contrast, in 37 prospective patients with CVT recanalization of occluded dural sinuses was frequently observed as early as 22 days after diagnosis using MRI; however, even early recanalization was not associated with the outcome [22]. This highlights the importance of hemodynamic factors for the long-term outcome of CVT, which cannot be assessed by current routine CTA and MRA.

In individual cases, a sudden increase in venous flow velocities concurrent with new clinical symptoms has been observed in the acute phase of illness when anticoagulation had to be stopped because of bleeding complications [15]. Flow velocities decreased again upon reinitiation of anticoagulation. However, currently it is not clear whether venous transcranial ultrasound can play a useful role in monitoring and steering anticoagulation in CVT.

References

1 Stolz E, Rahimi A, Gerriets T, Kraus J, Kaps M: Cerebral venous thrombosis: an all or nothing disease? Prognostic factors and long-term outcome. Clin Neurol Neurosurg 2005;107:99–107.

2 Ferro JM, Canhao P, Stam J, Bousser MG, Barinagarrementeria F: Prognosis of cerebral vein and dural sinus thrombosis: results of the International Study on Cerebral Vein and Dural Sinus Thrombosis (ISCVT). Stroke 2004;35:664–670.

3 Kosinski CM, Mull M, Schwarz M, Koch B, Biniek R, Schläfer J, Milkereit E, Willmes K, Schiefer J: Do normal D-dimer levels reliably exclude cerebral sinus thrombosis? Stroke 2004;35:2820–2825.
4 Stolz E: Cerebral veins and sinuses; in Baumgartner RW (ed): Handbook on Neurovascular Ultrasound. Front Neurol Neurosci, Basel, Karger, 2006, vol 21, pp 182–93.
5 Schreiber SJ, Stolz E, Valdueza JM: Transcranial ultrasonography of cerebral veins and sinuses. Eur J Ultrasound 2002;16:59–72.
6 Valdueza JM, Schmierer K, Mehraein S, Einhäupl KM: Assessment of normal flow velocity in basal cerebral veins: a transcranial Doppler ultrasound study. Stroke 1996;27:1221–1225.
7 Valdueza JM, Hoffmann O, Doepp F, Lehmann R, Einhäupl KM: Venous Doppler ultrasound assessment of parasellar region. Cerebrovasc Dis 1998;8:113–117.
8 Doepp F, Hoffmann O, Lehmann R, Einhäupl KM, Valdueza JM: The inferior petrosal sinus: assessment by transcranial Doppler ultrasound using the suboccipital approach. J Neuroimaging 1999;9:193–197.
9 Aaslid R, Lindegaard KF, Sorteberg W, Nornes H: Cerebral autoregulation dynamics in humans. Stroke 1989;20:45–52.
10 Rosengarten B, Rüskes D, Mendes I, Stolz E: A sudden arterial blood pressure decrease is compensated by an increase in intracranial blood volume. J Neurol 2002;249:538–541.
11 Stolz E, Kaps M, Kern A, Dorndorf W: Frontal bone windows for transcranial color-coded duplex sonography. Stroke 1999;30:814–820.
12 Baumgartner RW, Nirkko AC, Muri RM, Gonner F: Transoccipital power-based color-coded duplex sonography of cerebral sinuses and veins. Stroke 1997;28:1319–1323.
13 Stolz E, Babacan SS, Bodeker RH, Gerriets T, Kaps M: Interobserver and intraobserver reliability of venous transcranial color-coded flow velocity measurements. J Neuroimaging 2001;11: 385–392.
14 Wardlaw JM, Vaughan GT, Steers AJ, Sellar RJ: Transcranial Doppler ultrasound findings in cerebral venous sinus thrombosis. Case report. J Neurosurg 1994;80:332–335.
15 Valdueza JM, Schultz M, Harms L, Einhäupl KM: Venous transcranial Doppler ultrasound monitoring in acute dural sinus thrombosis. Report of two cases. Stroke 1995;26:1196–1199.
16 Ries S, Steinke W, Neff KW, Hennerici M: Echocontrast-enhanced transcranial color-coded sonography for the diagnosis of transverse sinus venous thrombosis. Stroke 1997;28:696–700.
17 Delcker A, Haussermann P, Weimar C: Effect of echo contrast media on the visualization of transverse sinus thrombosis with transcranial 3-D duplex sonography. Ultrasound Med Biol 1999;25:1063–1068.
18 Stolz E, Kaps M, Dorndorf W: Assessment of intracranial venous hemodynamics in normal individuals and patients with cerebral venous thrombosis. Stroke 1999;30:70–75.
19 Doepp F, Schreiber SJ, von Munster T, Rademacher J, Klingebiel R, Valdueza JM: How does the blood leave the brain? A systematic ultrasound analysis of cerebral venous drainage patterns. Neuroradiology 2004;46:565–570.
20 Valdueza JM, von Munster T, Hoffman O, Schreiber S, Einhaupl KM: Postural dependency of the cerebral venous outflow. Lancet 2000;355:200–201.
21 Stolz E, Gerriets T, Bodeker RH, Hugens-Penzel M, Kaps M: Intracranial venous hemodynamics is a factor related to a favorable outcome in cerebral venous thrombosis. Stroke 2002;33: 1645–1650.
22 Stolz E, Trittmacher S, Rahimi A, Gerriets T, Röttger C, Siekmann R, Kaps M: Influence of recanalization on outcome in dural sinus thrombosis: a prospective study. Stroke 2004;35: 544–547.
23 Stolz E, Kaps M, Kern A, Babacan SS, Dorndorf W: Transcranial color-coded duplex sonography of intracranial veins and sinuses in adults. Reference data from 130 volunteers. Stroke 1999;30: 1070–1075.
24 Baumgartner RW, Gonner F, Arnold M, Muri RM: Transtemporal power- and frequency-based color-coded duplex sonography of cerebral veins and sinuses. AJNR Am J Neuroradiol 1997;18: 1771–1781.
25 Baumgartner RW, Nirkko AC, Muri RM, Gonner F: Transoccipital power-based color-coded duplex sonography of cerebral sinuses and veins. Stroke 1997;28:1319–1323.

26 Doepp F, Hoffmann O, Lehmann R, Einhaupl KM, Valdueza JM: The inferior petrosal sinus: assessment by transcranial Doppler ultrasound using the suboccipital approach. J Neuroimaging 1999;9:193–197.
27 Canhão P, Batista P, Ferro JM: Venous transcranial Doppler in acute dural sinus thrombosis. J Neurol 1998;245:276–279.
28 Valdueza JM, Hoffmann O, Weih M, Mehraein S, Einhäupl KM: Monitoring of venous hemodynamics in patients with cerebral venous thrombosis by transcranial Doppler ultrasound. Arch Neurol 1999;56:229–234.

Erwin Stolz, MD, PhD
Department of Neurology, Justus Liebig University
Am Steg 14
DE–35385 Giessen (Germany)
Tel. +49 641 792 657, Fax +49 641 992 4509
E-Mail erwin.stolz@neuro.med.uni-giessen.de

Caso V, Agnelli G, Paciaroni M (eds): Handbook on Cerebral Venous Thrombosis.
Front Neurol Neurosci. Basel, Karger, 2008, vol 23, pp 122–131

Cerebral Venous Thrombosis in Newborns, Infants and Children

Jerome Y. Yager, Karina Black, Mary Bauman, Patricia Massicotte

Department of Pediatrics, Stollery Children's Hospital, University of Alberta, Edmonton, Alta., Canada

Abstract

Cerebral venous thrombosis is currently thought to be a relatively rare and benign entity in childhood. Recent studies however have shown that cerebral venous thrombosis is more common than previously believed, and carries significant mortality and neurologic morbidity. Neonates are the most commonly affected age group, compared to children >1 month of age. Magnetic resonance imaging venography is the gold standard by which this diagnosis should be made. Clinical trials are currently necessary to determine the most efficacious, safe, and age-specific approach for anticoagulation for this childhood disorder.

Copyright © 2008 S. Karger AG, Basel

Thrombosis of the cerebral venous system is recognized as a relatively rare, though highly underdiagnosed cause of stroke in newborns, infants and children [1–3]. Few studies have determined the population-based incidence of cerebral venous thrombosis (CVT) in children. Work done by the Canadian Pediatric Stroke Registry, however, estimated the incidence to be 0.67 per 100,000 per year, with a preponderance of neonates (43%), and over half (54%) being <1 year of age [2]. Interestingly, there appears to be a male predominance in this age group, with as many as 75% of neonates presenting with CVT being male [4].

Beyond the neonatal period, the incidence of CVT is relatively evenly distributed among the age groups to 18 years, and averages between 2 and 4% per year. Clinical presentation, however, as well as underlying etiologies, differ dramatically between the neonate and older infants and children [3, 5]. Diagnostic criteria, imaging modalities, and a menu of appropriate investigations have not been established in the pediatric population. In large part, this may be due to the absence of accepted standardized guidelines for treatment, and the criteria around which these might occur.

Table 1. Clinical presentation of CVT in neonates, infants and children

Presenting symptoms and signs	Neonate	Non-neonate
Seizures	+++	++
Diffuse neurologic manifestations	+++	++++
Decreased LOC	++	++
Headache	−−	+++
Irritability	+	+
None	++	+
Focal neurologic manifestations	+	++
Hemiparesis	+	++
Cranial nerve abnormalities	+	++
Visual deficit	−−	+
Speech impairment	−−	+
None	+++	++
Systemic manifestations		
Fever	−−	++
Poor feeding	++	+
Apnea	+	−−

The above table is a compilation of data from references [2, 5, 7]. The plus signs reflect the general incidence of presenting signs or symptoms in the neonate or non-neonatal age range. ++++ = ≥75%; +++ = ≥50%; ++ = ≥25%; + = ≥0%.

Outcomes appear better for children with CVT than for arterial ischemic stroke [6], though few studies have looked at long-term outcome, which suggests that current data underestimate the degree of neurologic morbidity associated with venous thrombosis in children.

The following chapter will highlight the known information regarding CVT in the newborn, infant and child, and attempt to propose a logical approach to these patients, with a look to the future research needed to improve our care of this underdiagnosed entity.

Clinical Presentation

Presentation of CVT differs between the newborn, and the infant and child greater than a month of age [2, 3, 5, 7] (table 1). In the newborn, both diffuse and focal symptoms present less frequently than they do in the infant and child. Frequently presenting features in the <1 month old are those of a neonatal encephalopathy, particularly lethargy or irritability, and poor feeding, with seizures being reported as the most common phenotype in 50–70% of babies. This is frequently associated with jitteriness, hypotonia, and apnea. In the older child, symptoms are more often of a chronic nature, with headache, drowsiness and lethargy being present in approximately half of the children, followed by vomiting and seizures. Fever, as a presenting sign occurs in 45% followed by focal signs of hemiparesis and cranial nerve abnormalities. The lack of features in the neonate especially, make the diagnosis difficult to establish, and likely is responsible for the underestimation of this entity in this age group.

Pathophysiology

Risk factors that predispose to the development of CVT also differ between the newborn and older child [1, 2, 7–9]. In this regard, the neonate may be at risk for CVT on the basis of intrauterine maternal or fetal factors, perinatal distress, or postpartum neonatal conditions. Wu et al. [7] describe 30 neonates seen over an 11-year period of time at a tertiary care facility in northern California. All patients, but one, were born at term. Maternal complications were present in 40% of the newborns, with chorioamnionitis being present in half of these (20%), followed by hypertension and diabetes in the mother accounting for 10% each. Perinatal distress including meconium, low 5-min Apgar score, and intubation at birth was present in almost 60% of the neonates with CVT. Neonatal medical complications occurred in 67%. Congenital heart disease was the most common and accounted for a third, followed by sepsis and disseminated intravascular coagulation, polycythemia and severe dehydration. Thirteen percent of the newborns had no identified risk factor. However, the majority had multiple risk factors for the development of CVT.

The Canadian Pediatric Stroke Registry has reported on the largest cohort of patients with CVT [2]. In this study, deVeber and the 16 included Canadian Tertiary pediatric centers found 160 patients with CVT over 6 years of enrollment. In this study, there was a very significant difference in the risk factors associated with CVT between neonates and non-neonates. As described in the above study, multiple risk factors frequently occurred in both age groups. Head and neck infections were particularly common in the older children, accounting for 38%, but only 16% in neonates. Acute systemic illnesses were more common in the neonate (84%), and again included perinatal complications, dehydration and sepsis, in the majority. In the non-neonates, chronic systemic disease occurred more often (60%), and included connective tissue disorders, hematologic abnormalities, cancer, cardiac disease, and disorders requiring an indwelling catheter. Interestingly, this study further highlighted the presence of prothrombotic disorders in all age groups (41%), though it was found to be twice as common in the non-neonate. The most frequent abnormality was the presence of anticardiolipin antibody. Other findings included decreased levels of protein C, antithrombin, and protein S. Much less frequent were abnormalities of fibrinogen, plasminogen, lupus anticoagulant, factor V Leiden and the G20210A prothrombin-gene mutation. The authors further found that in many of the cases related to protein C, S, and antithrombin, the disorder was likely acquired due to liver or kidney disease or sepsis. Others had received procoagulant drugs given during the course of cancer therapy, or as birth control.

Sebire et al. [5] described 42 children with CVT. In their group of patients, 40% had previous illness (chronic disease) most as described above. In those who were previously well (60%), the vast majority had an acute illness, most of which were infectious in etiology (73%). Interestingly, this group of investigators found a very high incidence of ear infection, mastoiditis or sinusitis (49%).

Less well documented is the finding that iron deficiency is a common abnormality found in children with stroke, and is equally distributed among those patients with arterial ischemic stroke and those associated with cerebral sinovenous thrombosis [10, 11]. In this regard, Hartfield et al. [10] found a significant association of arterial or venous stroke in children who were less than 18 months of age, had a mild respiratory or gastrointestinal infection, and iron deficiency. The authors further pointed out that the vast majority of these patients, though iron deficient, were not anemic. Sebire et al. [5] documented similar findings, but also pointed out the importance of several of the hemoglobinopathies including sickle cell trait and disease, and the thalassemias. In each of these forms of inherited or acquired abnormalities, blood cell deformability is likely one of the main reasons for the predisposition to CVT, though other possibilities include an increase in coagulability due to thrombocytosis, in the case of iron deficiency.

Not commonly thought of in children is the use of contraceptives. Bousser and Kittner [12], reviewed 25 studies looking at the association of oral contraceptives and stroke. He concluded that high estrogen content of $>50\,\mu g$ increased the risk of all stroke types, and that this risk is increased if the use of contraceptives is associated with hypertension, smoking or migraine. Importantly, the risk for cerebral sinus thrombosis was increased with the use of oral contraceptives, even at low dose, with estrogen $<50\,\mu g$.

Diagnosis

Cerebral sinovenous thrombosis, though rare, is largely underdiagnosed [13]. Familiarity with the clinical presentation is essential to the ultimate diagnosis

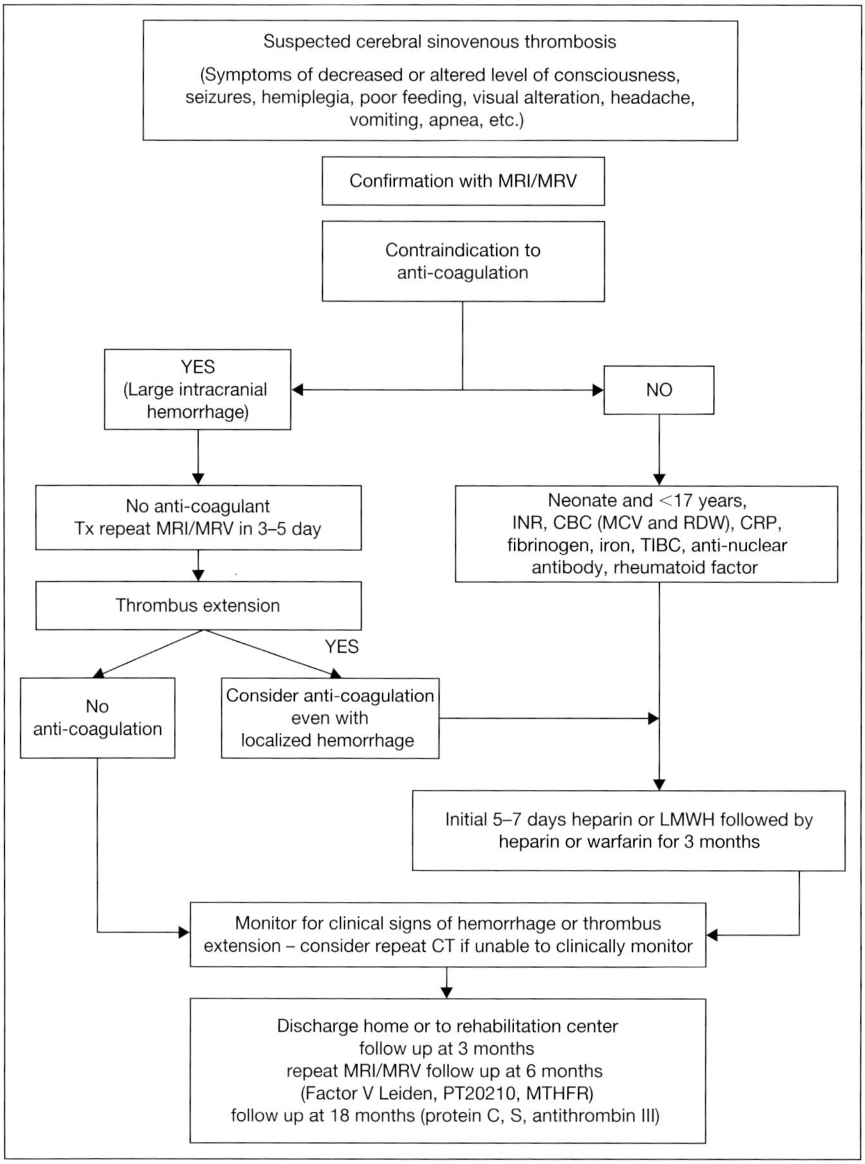

Fig. 1. Clinical pathway for the workup of CVT.

(table 1), and presents a challenge given its broad range of signs and symptoms, variable presentation being both acute and chronic, and ubiquity across age groups. The advent of neuroimaging has greatly improved the evaluation of children with suspected CSVT (fig. 1). Head ultrasonography is frequently used as a

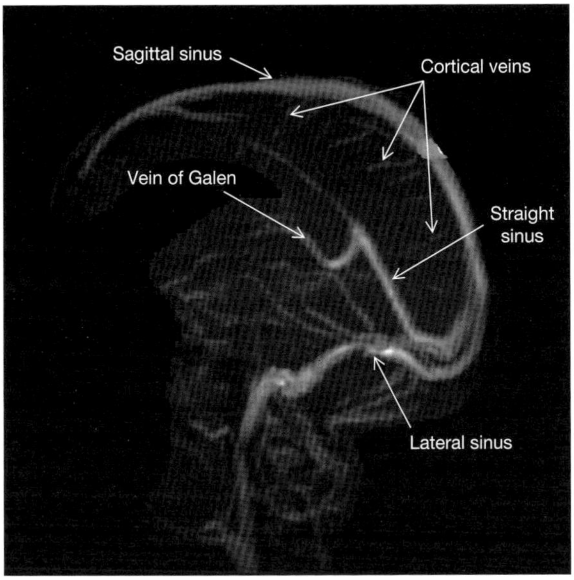

Fig. 2. MRV. Major venous sinuses are labeled with arrows.

screening tool in the diagnosis of brain injury of the newborn infant [14], but is no longer a consideration in the accurate visualization of CVT of the newborn. Computed tomography (CT) is certainly a rapid and effective method of detecting CVT, but not infrequently presents false-negative results [2]. Magnetic resonance imaging with venography (MRV) is clearly considered the gold standard technique to use in the diagnosis of CVT. Even in these circumstances however, experience is necessary to distinguish false-negative and false-positive results based on the timing of the image as it relates to the maturity of the clot and the presence of flow voids. Others, however, have certainly found CT venography to be as accurate in detection as MR venography [15–17].

The location of the clot and its attendant abnormalities are important, not only in the decision making process about treatment, but they also have significance related to prognosis and outcome (fig. 2). In this regard, pediatric studies have shown the superficial venous structures to be involved more frequently than deep venous structures, though the frequency of involvement between the two areas appears to be similar between the neonatal and nonneonatal age range. The superficial venous system is involved in the majority (85%), with over half of these involving the superior sagittal and lateral sinuses (55%). The deep venous system is involved less frequently (38%), with the straight and internal cerebral sinuses showing clot 24 and 10% of the time [2]. Clearly, multiple areas of involvement occurred frequently.

Infarction and hemorrhage were frequently seen in combination. Depending on publication, the combination appears in between 25% [1] and almost 60% [5] of patients, and may have a predilection for the newborn. Almost 1/3 of patients appear to have no evidence of parenchymal involvement, at least in newborns. These latter tend to present with seizures. Those children who have structural involvement of one or both hemispheres are more likely to be non-neonates, and to present with hemiparesis rather than seizures.

Treatment

The evidence for the treatment of CVT in children is clearly lacking as no clinical trials have been done comparing either no treatment to treatment, or anticoagulant therapies [18]. A review of 2 relatively small studies in the adult population did conclude that anticoagulant therapy for CVT was safe, and associated with an apparent reduction in the risk of death or dependency [19]. Still, further studies are required to evaluate the overall advantage of therapy versus the risk of hemorrhage.

The Hospital for Sick Children reviewed a cohort of 30 children with 32 episodes of CVT in the mid-1990s as part of an ongoing Canadian registry. Approximately one half of these children had systemic disease, the other 17 were previously healthy (10 non-neonates; 7 neonates). Of the 32, 10 children received standard heparin, and 12 children received low-molecular-weight heparin (LMWH). Eighteen children were treated for 3 months after the initial therapy, and 4 continued to receive LMWH for the duration of therapy. None of the children in the LMWH group had hemorrhagic transformation, though 1 child had a silent bleed with standard heparin therapy. The authors concluded that the use of anticoagulant therapy, particularly LMWH, for the treatment of childhood SVT was safe, thought clearly further studies were warranted [20].

Guidelines have been published, both in the UK and North America, based on the current best available evidence, though the latter is admittedly slim [21]. For newborns, the UK guidelines do not address treatment. The *Chest* guidelines [22] indicate that there is 2C evidence for the use of unfractionated or LMW heparin initially, and LMWH for 3 months in the newborn with documented CVT. In the case of large infarctions or a significant hemorrhagic component, the suggestion is for close radiographic monitoring, and treatment if there is extension, in the absence of further hemorrhage. For older children (>1 month of age), the recommendation in the UK guidelines is for the use of anticoagulation until recanalization or 6 months. Monagle et al. [22], in the *Chest* supplement again recommend unfractionated heparin or LMWH for 5–7 days, followed by LMWH or warfarin for 3–6 months. The same is recommended even in the presence of a reasonably small localized hemorrhagic transformation. New *Chest* guidelines will be published in the very near future, though to date, there have yet to be additional clinical trials in the use of anticoagulation for childhood CVT. In our own institution, the chest guidelines are currently followed. Asymptomatic CVT, found on routine imaging is generally not treated. Similarly, if there is significant hemorrhage involving >30% of a hemisphere, we will empirically not treat with anticoagulation. These children will be followed by serial cranial CT or magnetic resonance imaging, and if there is evidence of extension of the infarct and associated symptoms, treatment will be initiated.

Outcome

Information regarding the outcome of stroke in children is only now becoming available, in large part due the much enhanced recognition of this as an important contributor to morbidity and mortality in childhood. Outcomes in 163 patients, of whom 38 had SVT, with a distribution of 1/3 male and 2/3 female were reported by deVeber et al. [6] in 2000. The mean duration of follow-up was 2.0 years. In both the neonatal and non-neonatal groups, 80% were normal or had only mild deficits. The additional 20% were diagnosed as having moderate to severe deficits. Outcomes were better in CVT compared with outcomes in arterial ischemic strokes. Within the CVT group, neonates did somewhat better than did older children.

In the study conducted by Sebire et al. [5], of 42 non-neonates with CVT, 5 patients died, 1 due to recurrence, and the other 4 due to severe neurologic deficit. Of the survivors, 1/3 were reported as being normal. Twelve patients had symptoms of pseudotumor cerebri, and 14 of the children had cognitive difficulties. The findings appeared more suggestive of neurologic morbidity than did those reported by deVeber et al. [6]. Similar findings were reported by Carvalho et al. [1], who found no sequelae in 25 and 50% of neonates versus non-neonates. In a further comparison of neonates versus non-neonates, developmental delay occurred in 58 and 17%, sixth nerve deficit in 0 and 17%, hemiparesis in 0 and 8%, learning disability in 5 and 0%, and cortical visual deficit in 0 and 8%, respectively. Their reported mortality was 10% in neonates and 17% in older children. Length of follow-up was a mean of 22 months.

In each of the studies, a predisposing neurologic deficit predicted worse outcome. Other variables that provided some predictive value for worse outcome in these studies include the presence of an ischemic insult and multiple areas of involvement. All studies had relatively short duration to the determination of outcomes. In this regard, it is clear that as with many of the insults seen in the newborn and young child, we can expect to see the neurologic morbidity for CVT increase as reporting of long-term outcomes, particularly into school age, begin to surface.

Future Considerations

Currently, the best available data suggest that the incidence of cerebral venous sinus thrombosis is approximately 0.67 per 100,000. However, it is clear to those of us who work in the fields of neonatology and pediatric neurology, that this is likely a highly underestimated value. Moreover, the data currently available tell us that CVT is not the benign entity it was perhaps once thought to be. With current mortality rates approaching 10%, and neurologic morbidity in the range of 25 to over 50%, this is a disorder which can no longer be ignored. More so, given the fact that many of the underlying etiologies can be treated, and the advent of safe and efficacious anticoagulant therapy appears to be available. In this regard, future studies should direct themselves to the determination of those interventions (anticoagulation) which are age specific and most beneficial for neuroprotection, and diminished propagation of cerebral thrombus in childhood.

References

1 Carvalho KS, Bodensteiner JB, Connolly PJ, Garg BP: Cerebral venous thrombosis in children. J Child Neurol 2001;16:574–580.
2 deVeber G, Andrew M, Adams C, et al: Cerebral sinovenous thrombosis in children. N Engl J Med 2001;345:417–423.
3 Fitzgerald KC, Williams LS, Garg BP, Carvalho KS, Golomb MR: Cerebral sinovenous thrombosis in the neonate. Arch Neurol 2006;63:405–409.
4 Golomb MR, Dick PT, MacGregor DL, Curtis R, Sofronas M, deVeber GA: Neonatal arterial ischemic stroke and cerebral sinovenous thrombosis are more commonly diagnosed in boys. J Child Neurol 2004;19:493–497.
5 Sebire G, Tabarki B, Saunders DE, et al: Cerebral venous sinus thrombosis in children: risk factors, presentation, diagnosis and outcome. Brain 2005;128:477–489.
6 deVeber GA, MacGregor D, Curtis R, Mayank S: Neurologic outcome in survivors of childhood arterial ischemic stroke and sinovenous thrombosis. J Child Neurol 2000;15:316–324.
7 Wu YW, Miller SP, Chin K, et al: Multiple risk factors in neonatal sinovenous thrombosis. Neurology 2002;59:438–440.
8 Barron TF, Gusnard DA, Zimmerman RA, Clancy RR: Cerebral venous thrombosis in neonates and children. Pediatr Neurol 1992;8:112–116.
9 Bousser MG, Ferro JM: Cerebral venous thrombosis: an update. Lancet Neurol 2007;6:162–170.
10 Hartfield DS, Lowry NJ, Keene DL, Yager JY: Iron deficiency: a cause of stroke in infants and children. Pediatr Neurol 1997;16:50–53.
11 Yager JY, Hartfield DS: Neurologic manifestations of iron deficiency in childhood. Pediatr Neurol 2002;27:85–92.
12 Bousser MG, Kittner SJ: Oral contraceptives and stroke. Cephalalgia 2000;20:183–189.

13 Fink JN, McAuley DL: Cerebral venous sinus thrombosis: a diagnostic challenge. Intern Med J 2001;31:384–390.
14 Ment LR, Bada HS, Barnes P, et al: Practice parameter: neuroimaging of the neonate: report of the Quality Standards Subcommittee of the American Academy of Neurology and the Practice Committee of the Child Neurology Society. Neurology 2002;58:1726–1738.
15 Smith R, Hourihan MD: Investigating suspected cerebral venous thrombosis. BMJ 2007;334: 794–795.
16 Teasdale E: Cerebral venous thrombosis: making the most of imaging. J R Soc Med 2000;93: 234–237.
17 Khandelwal N, Agarwal A, Kochhar R, et al: Comparison of CT venography with MR venography in cerebral sinovenous thrombosis. AJR Am J Roentgenol 2006;187:1637–1643.
18 Chan AK, Deveber G, Monagle P, Brooker LA, Massicotte PM: Venous thrombosis in children. J Thromb Haemost 2003;1:1443–1455.
19 Stam J, de Bruijn S, deVeber G: Anticoagulation for cerebral sinus thrombosis. Stroke 2003;34: 1054–1055.
20 deVeber G, Chan A, Monagle P, et al: Anticoagulation therapy in pediatric patients with sinovenous thrombosis: a cohort study. Arch Neurol 1998;55:1533–1537.
21 DeVeber G: In pursuit of evidence-based treatments for paediatric stroke: the UK and Chest guidelines. Lancet Neurol 2005;4:432–436.
22 Monagle P, Chan A, Massicotte P, Chalmers E, Michelson AD: Antithrombotic therapy in children: the Seventh ACCP Conference on Antithrombotic and Thrombolytic Therapy. Chest 2004;126 (suppl 3):645S–687S.

Jerome Y. Yager, MD
Professor and Head, Section of Pediatric Neurosciences
Department of Pediatrics, 8213 Aberhart Centre 1
11402 University Avenue NW
Edmonton, Alta., T6G 2J3 (Canada)
Tel. +1 780 407 2064, Fax +1 780 407 8283, E-Mail jyager@ualberta.ca

Caso V, Agnelli G, Paciaroni M (eds): Handbook on Cerebral Venous Thrombosis.
Front Neurol Neurosci. Basel, Karger, 2008, vol 23, pp 132–143

Treatment of Cerebral Venous and Sinus Thrombosis

F. Masuhr, K. Einhäupl

Department of Neurology, Charité – Universitätsmedizin Berlin, Berlin, Germany

Abstract

Cerebral venous and sinus thrombosis (CVST) is a rather rare disease which accounts for less than 1% of all strokes. Current therapeutic measures which are used in clinical practice include the use of anticoagulants such as dose-adjusted intravenous heparin or body weight-adjusted subcutaneous low molecular weight heparin, the use of thrombolysis, and symptomatic therapy including control of seizures and elevated intracranial pressure. We reviewed the strength of evidence reported in the literature to support these interventions and provide treatment recommendations based on the best available evidence. Patients with CVST without contraindications for anticoagulation (AC) should be treated either with body weight-adjusted subcutaneous low molecular weight heparin or dose-adjusted intravenous heparin. Concomitant intracranial hemorrhage related to CVST is not a contraindication for heparin therapy. The optimal duration of oral AC after the acute phase is unclear. Oral AC may be given for 3 months if CVST was secondary to a transient risk factor, for 6–12 months in patients with idiopathic CVST and in those with 'mild' hereditary thrombophilia. Indefinite AC should be considered in patients with two or more episodes of CVST and in those with one episode of CVST and 'severe' hereditary thrombophilia. There is insufficient evidence to support the use of either systemic or local thrombolysis in patients with CVST. If patients deteriorate despite adequate AC and other causes of deterioration have been ruled out, thrombolysis may be a therapeutic option in selected cases, possibly in those without intracranial hemorrhage. There are no controlled data about the risks and benefits of certain therapeutic measures to reduce an elevated intracranial pressure (with brain displacement) in patients with severe CVST. Antiedema treatment (including hyperventilation, osmotic diuretics, craniectomy) should be used as life-saving interventions.

Copyright © 2008 S. Karger AG, Basel

Cerebral venous and sinus thrombosis (CVST) accounts for less than 1% of all strokes. Diagnosis is still frequently overlooked or delayed due to the wide spectrum of clinical symptoms and the often subacute or lingering onset. Early diagnosis is crucial since anticoagulation (AC) may reduce the risk of a fatal outcome and severe disability without promoting intracranial hemorrhage.

The following chapter provides treatment recommendations for patients with CVST based on the best available evidence from the current literature [1].

Treatment

Available treatment data from controlled trials favor the use of AC in patients with CVST because it may reduce the risk of a fatal outcome and severe disability and does not promote ICH [2, 3]. In the prospective study of Einhäupl et al. [2] which compared dose-adjusted intravenous heparin with placebo in 20 patients, 8 patients in the heparin group recovered completely and none died, whereas only 1 patient in the placebo group recovered fully and 3 patients died. Three patients with previous ICH recovered completely and no new hemorrhages occurred in the heparin group, whereas in the placebo group 2 patients with pretreatment ICH died and 2 new hemorrhages were observed.

The only other randomized trial compared body weight-adjusted subcutaneous low molecular weight heparin (LMWH) with placebo in 60 patients with CVST [3]. A poor outcome – defined as death or Barthel index <15 – was observed after 3 weeks in 6 of the 30 patients treated with LMWH (20%) compared to 7 of the 29 controls (24%). After 12 weeks, 3 patients (10%) in the LMWH group and 6 patients (21%) in the placebo group had a poor outcome, which corresponds to a nonsignificant absolute risk reduction of 11% in favor of the active treatment. No new ICH or secondary worsening of the 15 patients with pretreatment hemorrhage was observed in the LMWH group. A meta-analysis of these two trials showed that the use of AC led to an absolute risk reduction in death or dependency of 13% (confidence interval −30 to +3%) with a relative risk reduction of 54% [4]. Although this difference is not statistically significant (presumably due to the small sample size with a total of 79 patients), both trials show a consistent and clinically meaningful trend in favor of AC and demonstrate the safety of anticoagulant therapy. However, it is unclear, whether treatment with full-dose intravenous heparin or subcutaneously applied LMWH is equally effective. We recommend the use of intravenous heparin particularly in critically ill patients because the activated partial thromboplastin time (aPTT) may normalize within 1 h after discontinuation of the infusion if complications occur or surgical intervention is necessary. In patients with isolated intracranial hypertension (and proven CVST) and threatened vision with the need for repeated lumbar punctures to remove cerebrospinal fluid (CSF) in order to obtain a normal closing pressure, AC should be withheld until 24 h after the last lumbar puncture [1].

There is currently no evidence from randomized controlled trials about the efficacy and safety of either systemic or local thrombolytic therapy in patients with CVST. Thrombolytic therapy has the potential to provide faster restitution of venous outflow and positive effects of local thrombolytic treatment of CVST have increasingly been reported from uncontrolled series [5–8]. Patients were either treated with heparin and urokinase or heparin and recombinant tissue plasminogen activator (rtPA) which may carry less bleeding complications due to its clot selectiveness and shorter half-life. Two uncontrolled studies which used rtPA in combination with dose-adjusted intravenous heparin included a total of 21 patients [6, 7]. In the Korean study [6] which included 9 patients, a mean total dose of 135 mg (range 50–300 mg) rtPA was used compared to 46 mg (range 23–128 mg) in the American study [7] which included 12 patients. Both studies placed a microcatheter directly into the thrombus via the transfemoral vein and performed a bolus injection of rtPA followed by continuous infusion. In the two studies combined, rapid (mean time of 20 h in the Korean and 29 h in the American study) and complete recanalization was achieved in 15 of 21 patients and 14 of 21 patients showed a complete clinical recovery. However, there were two extracerebral bleeding complications in the Korean study and 2 patients with pretreatment ICH in the American study worsened because of increased intracerebral bleeding which required surgery in one case. Thus, although recanalization was rapidly achieved, local thrombolysis may carry a higher risk of bleeding complications compared to AC particularly if pretreatment ICH is present [9]. Controlled trials which compare heparin therapy and local thrombolysis are lacking and there is no evidence that clinical outcome is better than with heparin alone. Currently, local thrombolysis may be a therapeutic option for patients at high risk for a poor outcome despite heparin therapy. The International Study on Cerebral Vein and Dural Sinus Thrombosis (ISCVT) identified coma on admission and thrombosis of the deep venous system apart from underlying causes as the most important predictors for a poor clinical outcome [10]. More than 80% of the included 624 adult patients were treated with AC. Comatose patients may define a subgroup of patients with CVST who are at high risk of death despite AC [11]. Under this particular condition, the effect of AC may come too late to prevent irreversible brain damage and these patients may possibly benefit from thrombolytic therapy. A published systematic review on the use of thrombolytics in CVST suggested a possible benefit in such severe cases [12]. Thirty-eight of the reported patients were comatose at the start of thrombolytic therapy, 6 (13%) of whom died. Intracranial hemorrhage occurred in 17% and was associated with clinical deterioration in 5% of cases. In comparison, a retrospective analysis found that 53% of patients with stupor or coma at the start of dose-adjusted intravenous heparin therapy died [11]. In the ISCVT, 38.7% of the comatose patients died [10]. However, the results of the review were based on case reports and uncontrolled case series, and there are yet no established clinical criteria for the use of thrombolytics in CVST. If patients deteriorate despite adequate AC and other causes of deterioration have been ruled out, thrombolysis may be a therapeutic option in selected cases, possibly in those without intracranial hemorrhage [1]. A controlled randomized trial is warranted to further study the efficacy and safety of thrombolysis in CVST.

Pragmatic Therapy

Heparin Therapy

Dose-adjusted intravenous heparin treatment should be started immediately with a bolus of 3,000–5,000 IU after the diagnosis, even if a hemorrhagic infarct is present. The aPTT should at least be doubled. Continuous treatment using an intravenous infusion system is started with 1,000–1,200 IU per hour, followed by an increase of 100–200 IU per hour every 6–8 h until aPTT is doubled. The required heparin dosage varies significantly among patients but administration of very high dosages (>2,000–3,000 IU/h) may reflect antithrombin III deficiency or wrong filling of the perfusion syringe since other causes of heparin resistance are rare. Alternatively, LMWH (e.g. nadroparin in a dose of 180 antifactor Xa U/kg/24 h administered by two subcutaneous injections daily) can be given particularly in uncomplicated cases. A meta-analysis which compared the efficacy of fixed dose subcutaneous LMWH versus adjusted dose unfractionated heparin for extracerebral venous thromboembolism found a superiority for LMWH and significantly less major bleeding complications [13]. Further advantages of LMWH include the route of administration which increases the mobility of patients and the lack of laboratory monitoring and subsequent dose adjustments. Heparin therapy should be continued until remission of the acute stage of the disease (normalizing level of consciousness or remission of mental confusion, improvement of headache and focal neurological deficits).

Oral AC

After the acute stage, therapy is switched over to oral AC. Three tablets (à 3 mg per tablet) are given as a single dose on the 1st day of phenprocoumon therapy, followed by 2 tablets on the 2nd and 3rd day. Further dosage is depending on the actual international normalized ratio (INR) value with a target INR of 2.0–3.0. Effective AC must be ensured during adjustment to coumarin or warfarin therapy. This is accomplished by continuing full-dose heparin therapy until the INR value is in its target range. If deterioration of the clinical status appears, heparin therapy should be resumed without termination of oral AC, because deterioration is usually due to ineffective AC during coumarin or warfarin adjustment. However, oral AC should be stopped if clinical deterioration continues. If CVST occurs during pregnancy, oral AC should be avoided due to its possible teratogenic effect and ability to pass the placenta. In these cases, AC should be continued with heparin. However, placenta hemorrhage with subsequent placenta insufficiency may also appear during heparin therapy.

Controlled data about the benefit and optimal duration of oral AC in patients with CVST do not exist. An MRI follow-up study of 33 patients suggested that recanalization occurs within the first 4 months after CVST irrespective of further AC [14]. These data may provide some guidance on the optimal duration of AC but whether incomplete or absent recanalization increases the risk of recurrence is not known. In this as well as in the study by Strupp et al. [15], no relapses occurred during follow-up time although more than 40% of the patients had incomplete or no recanalization.

Analogous to patients with extracerebral venous thrombosis, oral AC with a target INR of 2.0–3.0 may be given for 3 months if CVST was secondary to a transient (reversible) risk factor and for 6–12 months if it was idiopathic [16]. However, the risk of recurrence of CVST may be lower than that of extracerebral venous thrombosis. In the ISCVT, 2.2% of all patients had a recurrent sinus thrombosis with a median follow-up of 16 months [10] and prolonged AC may expose some patients to an unnecessary bleeding risk, although there was also a risk of 4.3% for other thrombotic events during follow-up including 2.5% of pelvic or limb venous thrombosis and 0.5% of pulmonary embolism.

Oral AC is also recommended for 6–12 months in patients with extracerebral venous thrombosis and a 'mild' hereditary thrombophilia such as protein C and S deficiency, heterozygous factor V Leiden or prothrombin G20210A mutations. Long-term treatment should be considered for patients with a 'severe' hereditary thrombophilia which carries a high risk of recurrence, such as antithrombin deficiency, homozygous factor V Leiden mutation, or two or more thrombophilic conditions. Indefinite AC is also recommended in patients with two or more episodes of idiopathic objectively documented extracerebral venous thrombosis [16]. Thus, in the absence of controlled data the decision on the duration of anticoagulant therapy must be based on individual hereditary and precipitating factors as well as on the potential bleeding risks of long-term AC. Regular follow-up visits should be performed after termination of AC and patients should be informed about early signs (headache) indicating a possible relapse.

Symptomatic Therapy

Symptomatic therapy includes the use of antiepileptic drugs (AED), management of increased intracranial pressure (ICP), the control of psychomotor agitation and psychotic features if present, analgesic treatment (table 1) and the use of antibiotics in patients with septic CVST.

Table 1. Treatment strategies for CVST

Substance	Indication	Aim	Dosage	Duration
Heparin	During the acute stage	aPTT doubled	Bolus of 3,000–5,000 IU, then 1,000–1,500 IU (average 1,200 IU) per hour	Until clinical condition is stable (continuous stabilization of symptoms or complete remission, usually within 10–14 days)
LMWH (e.g. nadoparine)	During the acute stage	Body weight-adjusted therapeutic dose	180 antifactor Xa U/kg per 24 h	Until clinical condition is stable (continuous stabilization of symptoms or complete remission, usually within 10–14 days)
Phenprocoumon	Subacute stage	Target INR 2.0–3.0	1st day, 3 tablets 2nd and 3rd day, 2 tablets 4th day, according to INR values	6–12 months in idiopathic CVST, 6–12 months in patients with a coagulation disorder (see text)
Warfarin	Subacute stage	Target INR 2.0–3.0	Days 1 and 2, 10 mg/day 3rd day, according to INR values	6–12 months in idiopathic CVST, 6–12 months in patients with a coagulation disorder (see text)
Phenytoin	Prophylactic in patients at risk for seizures (see text) and in all patients after the first seizure	Avoidance of seizures during the acute stage in patients at risk and prevention of status epilepticus after the first seizure	500–1,000 mg intravenously over 4–6 h after the first seizure; for prophylaxis or after intravenous application: 300 mg tid orally	The duration of AED therapy should be based on an individual decision (see text)

Table 1. (continued)

Substance	Indication	Aim	Dosage	Duration
Acetaminophen	Mild headache	Necessary pain relief and justifiable sedation (assessment of neurological status)	500–1,000 mg tid	On demand
Tramadol	Severe headache	Necessary pain relief and justifiable sedation (assessment of neurological status)	50–100 mg tid orally or subcutaneously	On demand
Triflupromazine	Severe nausea and vomiting	Treatment of nausea with justifiable sedation	10–20 mg intravenously	As long as clinically necessary
Haloperidol	Agitation, psychotic symptoms	Treatment of agitation and psychosis with justifiable sedation	5–20 mg intravenously or orally	As long as clinically necessary
Midazolam	Sedation	Short-acting sedation for diagnostic or therapeutical procedures	5–10 mg intravenously	As long as clinically necessary
Mannitol 20%	Critical rise of ICP, threatening brain herniation	Reduction of ICP	125 ml intravenously over 10–15 min 4–6×/day, dose reduction by doubling the application intervals	Usually for 48–72 h and as long as serum osmolality is <320 mOsm/kg

Treatment of Seizures

The prophylactic use of AED in all patients with CVST is controversial. Whereas some authors recommend prophylactic treatment because of the high incidence of seizures (and series of seizures or even status epilepticus) and their possible detrimental effects on the metabolic situation during the acute phase of the disease [17], others restrict the use of anticonvulsants to patients with seizures [18]. Two studies identified focal sensory and motor deficits, the presence of parenchymal lesions and intracranial hemorrhage on admission CCT/MRI and cortical vein thrombosis as independent predictors of early symptomatic seizures [19, 20]. Although data are insufficient to give recommendations, these findings suggest that prophylactic treatment with AED may be a therapeutic option for those patients, whereas it is not warranted when there are no focal neurological deficits and no focal parenchymal lesions on brain scan (e.g. patients with isolated intracranial hypertension).

If no antiepileptic treatment has been performed before the first seizure occurs, effective concentrations of phenytoin should be achieved within 4–6 h because status epilepticus frequently occurs in patients with CVST and is associated with an increased mortality [20].

The risk of residual epilepsy after CVST is low compared to the high rate of patients with early seizures. Reported incidences range from 5 to 10.6% [10, 19, 21]. In a Portuguese series [19], all late seizures occurred within the 1st year. A hemorrhagic lesion in the acute brain scan was the strongest predictor of postacute seizures. In all series together, late seizures were more common in patients with early symptomatic seizures than in those patients with none. Thus, prolonged treatment with AED for 1 year may be reasonable for patients with early seizures and hemorrhagic lesions on admission brain scan, whereas in patients without these risk factors AED therapy may be tapered off gradually after the acute stage [see the chapter by Ferro and Canhão, this vol., pp. 161–171].

Treatment of Elevated ICP

Although brain swelling is observed in about 50% of all patients with CVST on CCT, minor brain edema needs no other treatment than AC which improves the venous outflow sufficiently to reduce ICP in most patients [18, 22]. In patients with isolated intracranial hypertension and threatened vision, a lumbar puncture with sufficient CSF removal to obtain a normal closing pressure should be performed before starting AC 24 h after the puncture. There are no controlled data but acetazolamide may be considered in patients with persistent papilloedema. In few patients, vision continues to deteriorate despite repeated lumbar punctures and/or acetazolamide. In these cases, shunting procedures (lumboperitoneal, ventriculoperitoneal shunts or optic nerve fenestration) should be considered [1].

Antiedematous treatment is necessary in only 20% of patients and should be carried out according to general principles of therapy of raised ICP (head elevation at about 30°, hyperventilation with a target $PaCO_2$ pressure of 30–35 mm Hg, intravenous application of osmotic diuretics). However, one should keep in mind that osmotic substances might be harmful in venous outflow obstruction since they are not as quickly eliminated from the intracerebral circulation as in other conditions. The use of tris-hydroxy-methyl-aminomethane which decreases ICP after intravenous administration via an alkalotic vasoconstriction may be a therapy option in ventilated patients. Restricted volume intake for treatment of brain edema must be avoided, since these measures can cause an additional deterioration of blood viscosity. Steroids can not be generally recommended for treatment of elevated ICP since their efficacy is unproven and they may be harmful through their promotion of the thrombotic process. No benefit of steroids was found in a case-control study of the ISCVT [23].

In severe cases with threatening transtentorial brain herniation due to a unilateral large hemorrhagic infarct, decompressive surgery may be the only way to save the patient's life. Local thrombolysis seems to be no treatment option in such cases because of the incalculable risk of further ICH extension with an additional detrimental effect on ICP. Stefini et al. [24] reported 3 patients with fixed dilated pupils due to transtentorial herniation who underwent decompressive surgery, 2 of whom recovered with only minor neurological sequelae. The hemorrhagic infarct should not be removed because neuronal damage is often less pronounced in CVST-related hemorrhage explaining the possible reversibility of even severe clinical symptoms [25].

Treatment of Septic CVST

Septic CVST almost always occurs in patients with bacterial cranial infections. The clinical signs of CVST are often accompanied or dominated by the symptoms of local infection, fever and a CSF pleocytosis due to an associated bacterial meningitis. Septic CVST is due to a contiguous propagation of thrombosis from infections of the nose, the ears or the neck. The cavernous sinus is more frequently affected by infections of the face, whereas the lateral and petrosal sinuses are more frequently affected by infections of the ear. A more distant focus is an exceptional cause [26]. Septic cavernous sinus thrombosis has a distinct clinical picture with chemosis, exophthalmos, and painful ophthalmoplegia (with lesions of the III, IV and VIth cranial nerves). It is initially unilateral but frequently spreads to the opposite site, whereas extension to other sinuses or to the intracavernous portion of the carotid artery is rare but often dramatic. Septic thrombosis of posterior sinuses often extends to other sinuses and veins of the brain, causing the same clinical features as noninfective CVST.

Isolated septic cortical vein thrombosis without affection of the sinus is extremely rare [27]. Clinical symptoms (meningeal syndrome, seizures and focal signs) will often be attributed to purulent meningitis and diagnosis will only be established if conventional angiography is performed.

Prognosis of septic CVST is worse compared to nonseptic cases with reported mortality rates ranging from 50 to 80%. Treatment includes the early administration of systemic antibiotics, surgical removal of the infectious focus and the use of AC. Antibiotics will be chosen according to the bacteria found after surgical removal, in the CSF, blood samples or in smear examinations. Treatment should be started with antibiotics which are highly effective against bacteria commonly found in infections of the face, neck or ear. We start with a third-generation cephalosporin (e.g. ceftriaxone 1×2 g/day intravenously) combined with a penicillinase-resistant penicillin (flucloxacillin 6×2 g/day intravenously). In patients with suspected nosocomial infection, meropenem (3×2 g/day intravenously) or ceftazidine (3×2 g/day intravenously) and vancomycin (4×0.5 g/day intravenously) are recommended. The effect of heparin in septic CVST has not been systematically investigated but most authors favor the use of heparin. We have had so far no hemorrhagic complications when AC was used in patients with septic CVST.

Recommendations

Patients with CVST without contraindications for AC should be treated either with body weight-adjusted subcutaneous LMWH or dose-adjusted intravenous heparin. Concomitant intracranial hemorrhage related to CVST is not a contraindication for heparin therapy. The optimal duration of oral AC after the acute phase is unclear. Oral AC may be given for 3 months if CVST was secondary to a transient risk factor, for 6–12 months in patients with idiopathic CVST and in those with 'mild' hereditary thrombophilia. Indefinite AC should be considered in patients with two or more episodes of CVST and in those with one episode of CVST and 'severe' hereditary thrombophilia.

There is insufficient evidence to support the use of either systemic or local thrombolysis in patients with CVST. If patients deteriorate despite adequate AC and other causes of deterioration have been ruled out, thrombolysis may be a therapeutic option in selected cases, possibly in those without intracranial hemorrhage. There are no controlled data about the risks and benefits of certain therapeutic measures to reduce an elevated ICP (with brain displacement) in patients with severe CVST. Antiedema treatment (including hyperventilation, osmotic diuretics, craniectomy) should be used as life-saving interventions.

References

1 Einhäupl K, Bousser MG, de Bruijn SFTM, Ferro JM, Martinelli M, Masuhr F, Stam J: EFNS guideline on the treatment of cerebral venous and sinus thrombosis. Eur J Neurol 2006;13:553–559.

2 Einhäupl KM, Villringer A, Meister W, Mehraein S, Garner C, Pellkofer M, Haberl RL, Pfister HW, Schmiedek P: Heparin treatment in sinus venous thrombosis. Lancet 1991;338:597–600.

3 De Bruijn SFTM, Stam J, for the Cerebral Venous Sinus Thrombosis Study Group: Randomized, placebo-controlled trial of anticoagulant treatment with low-molecular-weight heparin for cerebral sinus thrombosis. Stroke 1999;30:484–488.

4 Stam J, de Bruijn SFTM, deVeber G: Anticoagulation for cerebral sinus thrombosis. Cochrane Database Syst Rev 2001;4:CD002005.

5 Horowitz M, Purdy P, Unwin H, Carstens G, Greenlee R, Hise J, Kopitnik T, Batjer H, Rollins N, Samson D: Treatment of dural sinus thrombosis using selective catheterisation and urokinase. Ann Neurol 1995;38:58–67.

6 Kim SY, Suh JH: Direct endovascular thrombolytic therapy for dural sinus thrombosis: infusion of alteplase. Am J Neuroradiol 1997;18:639–645.

7 Frey IL, Muro GJ, McDougall CG, Dean BL, Jahnke HK: Cerebral venous thrombosis. Combined intrathrombus rtPA and intravenous heparin. Stroke 1999;30:489–494.

8 Wasay M, Bakshi R, Kojan S, Bobustuc G, Dubey N, Unwin DH: Nonrandomized comparison of local urokinase thrombolysis versus systemic heparin anticoagulation for superior sagittal sinus thrombosis. Stroke 2001;32:2310–2317.

9 Bousser MG: Cerebral venous thrombosis. Nothing, heparin, or local thrombolysis? Stroke 1999;30:481–483.

10 Ferro JM, Canhão P, Stam J, Bousser MG, Barinagarrementeria F, for the ISCVT Investigators: Prognosis of cerebral vein and dural sinus thrombosis. Results of the International Study on Cerebral Vein and Dural Sinus Thrombosis (ISCVT). Stroke 2004;35:664–670.

11 Mehraein S, Schmidtke K, Villringer A, Valdueza JM, Masuhr F: Heparin treatment in cerebral sinus and venous thrombosis: patients at risk of fatal outcome. Cerebrovasc Dis 2003;15:17–21.

12 Canhão P, Falcão F, Ferro JM: Thrombolytics for cerebral sinus thrombosis. A systematic review. Cerebrovasc Dis 2003;15:159–166.

13 Van Dongen CJJ, van den Belt AGM, Prins MH, Lensing AWA: Fixed dose subcutaneous low molecular weight heparins versus adjusted dose unfractionated heparin for venous thromboembolism. Cochrane Database Syst Rev 2004;4:CD001100.

14 Baumgartner RW, Studer A, Arnold M, Georgiadis D: Recanalisation of cerebral venous thrombosis. J Neurol Neurosurg Psychiatry 2003;74:459–461.

15 Strupp M, Covi M, Seelos K, Dichgans M, Brandt T: Cerebral venous thrombosis: correlation between recanalization and clinical outcome – a long-term follow-up of 40 patients. J Neurol 2002;249:1123–1124.

16 Büller HR, Agnelli G, Hull RH, Hyers TM, Prins MH, Raskob GE: Antithrombotic therapy for venous thromboembolic disease. The seventh ACCP conference on antithrombotic and thrombolytic therapy. Chest 2004;126:401S–428S.

17 Einhäupl KM, Masuhr F: Cerebral venous and sinus thrombosis – an update. Eur J Neurol 1994;1:109–126.

18 Ameri A, Bousser MG: Cerebral venous thrombosis. Neurol Clin 1992;10:87–111.

19 Ferro JM, Correia M, Rosas MJ, Pinto AN, Neves G, for the Cerebral Venous Thrombosis Portuguese Collaborative Study Group: Seizures in cerebral vein and dural sinus thrombosis. Cerebrovasc Dis 2003;15:78–83.

20 Masuhr F, Busch M, Amberger N, Ortwein H, Weih M, Neumann K, Einhäupl K, Mehraein S: Risk and predictors of early epileptic seizures in acute cerebral venous and sinus thrombosis. Eur J Neurol 2006;13:852–856.

21 Preter M, Tzourio C, Ameri A, Bousser MG: Long-term prognosis in cerebral venous thrombosis – follow-up of 77 patients. Stroke 1996;27:243–246.

22 Masuhr F, Mehraein S, Einhäupl K: Cerebral venous and sinus thrombosis. J Neurol 2004;251:11–23.

23 Canhão P, Cortesão A, Cabral M, Ferro J, Stam J, Bousser MG, Barinagarrementeria F, for the ISCVT Investigators: Are steroids useful for the treatment of cerebral venous thrombosis? ISCVT results. Cerebrovasc Dis 2004;17(suppl 5):16.
24 Stefini R, Latronico N, Cornali C, Rasulo F, Bollati A: Emergent decompressive craniectomy in patients with fixed dilated pupils due to cerebral venous and dural sinus thrombosis: report of three cases. Neurosurgery 1999;45:626–629.
25 Villringer A, Mehraein S, Einhäupl KM: Pathophysiological aspects of cerebral sinus venous thrombosis. J Neuroradiol 1994;21:72–80.
26 Southwick FS, Richardson EP, Swartz MN: Septic thrombosis of the dural venous sinuses. Medicine 1986;65:82–106.
27 Di Nubile MJ, Boom WH, Southwick FS: Septic cortical thrombophlebitis. J Infect Dis 1990;161: 1216–1220.

Prof. Dr. med. K. Einhäupl
Department of Neurology, Charité – Universitätsmedizin Berlin, Chariteplatz 1
DE–10117 Berlin (Germany)
Tel. +49 30 450 560 074, Fax +49 30 450 560 932, E-Mail Karl.Einhaeupl@charite.de

Caso V, Agnelli G, Paciaroni M (eds): Handbook on Cerebral Venous Thrombosis.
Front Neurol Neurosci. Basel, Karger, 2008, vol 23, pp 144–160

Interventional Neuroradiology in the Treatment of Cerebral Venous Thrombosis

Valeria Caso[a], *Antonia Maria Rosa Billeci*[a], *Didier Leys*[b]

[a]Stroke Unit and Division of Cardiovascular Medicine, Department of Internal Medicine, University of Perugia, Santa Maria della Misericordia Hospital, Sant' Andrea delle Fratte, Perugia, Italy; [b]Department of Neurology, Stroke Unit, University of Lille, Lille, France

Abstract

Heparin is the standard of care in cerebral venous thrombosis. Local thrombolysis is believed to better restore venous blood flow than heparin. Thrombolysis is also used when the patient's condition worsens despite heparin and symptomatic treatment. The most frequently described cause of worsening is inadequate anticoagulation. Clinical deterioration due to thrombosis progression in properly anticoagulated patients is rarely observed. When it is observed, thrombolytic treatment should be considered as a valid option. This is so, even in the absence of clear evidence from randomized trials that clinical outcome is superior. Furthermore, in theory, hemorrhagic risk is higher in thrombolysis compared to heparin, especially when a pretreatment hemorrhage is already present. Thus, this fear that hemorrhagic stroke can deteriorate due to thrombolysis treatment leads to the development of improved mechanical techniques that lower the risk of bleeding. One of these devices is rheolytic thrombectomy, which utilizes the Venturi effect which creates a negative pressure fragmenting and aspirating the cerebral venous thrombus. These devices can be utilized in combination with thrombolysis. The interventional neuroradiology data published until now are promising. However, whether interventional radiology is more effective or safer than heparin therapy even in patients who can be treated by heparin can only be answered by randomized controlled trials. There is no reason to recommend interventional radiology in these patients who are likely to have a good outcome unless proven superior in a trial.

Copyright © 2008 S. Karger AG, Basel

In patients with cerebral venous thrombosis (CVT), mortality rates declined over the last 30 years [1–5] as a consequence of: (a) earlier diagnosis with magnetic resonance imaging (MRI) [6]; (b) possibility to diagnose CVT in patients with isolated intracranial hypertension [7–9] or headache [3], who usually have a favorable outcome [4], and (c) policies of early anticoagulation [6, 10]. Although the level of evidence for its efficacy is not very high, heparin therapy is safe in CVT [4], even in hemorrhagic cases [6, 10, 11] and recommended as the standard therapy [6]. Interventional neuroradiology has been suggested as another therapeutic option [12].

The aim of this chapter is to evaluate using data from the literature the rationale for interventional neuroradiology in CVT, feasibility, efficacy and safety issues, and to make proposals for the future. The literature was limited to 5 languages: English (all authors), Italian and German (V.C.), French and Dutch (D.L.). The use of articles written in other languages was restricted to that of their English abstract.

Rationale for Interventional Neuroradiology in CVT

Heparin being the standard of care in CVT, the question of whether interventional neuroradiology should be used does not apply to those patients who are likely to tolerate heparin and to have a reasonable chance of good outcome under heparin. Therefore, it is crucial to identify predictors of outcome as soon as possible.

Factors identifiable at admission that have been found as associated with a poor short-term outcome are coma, intracerebral hemorrhage, delta sign on CT, central nervous system infection, focal deficits, symptoms of encephalopathy (generalized seizures, abulia, delirium, stupor or coma), bilateral pyramidal tract signs or deep location of the thrombosis (straight sinus or Galien vein) [3–9, 11, 13–16]. The outcome of deep CVT appears difficult to clearly identify; the criteria of bad outcome in these forms could be the presence of a coma and extreme ages of life [17, 18].

Factors associated at admission with a good short-term outcome are normal consciousness, absence of intracerebral hemorrhage or infarct, younger age, absence of signs of encephalopathy, isolated intracranial hypertension, absence of focal deficit, absence of cancer, and early heparin therapy [3–9, 11, 13–18].

However, most studies evaluating the outcome in CVT shared the following issues [3–9, 11, 13–18]: (a) a long period of recruitment leading to heterogeneity in the diagnostic work-up (especially in the radiological procedure), and treatment; (b) a retrospective design, leading to incomplete case ascertainment and underestimation of so-called 'minor sequelae'; (c) a recruitment bias with a high proportion of benign cases such as isolated intracranial hypertension; (d) the absence of multivariate analysis, or (e) evaluation in the setting of a drug trial, i.e. in a group of patients who are not representative of all patients with CVT, and are usually treated in highly specialized units.

Other therapeutic options, especially interventional radiology seem to be interesting options to be tested in patients who have predictors of poor outcome, and in the case of worsening despite appropriate anticoagulation.

Feasibility of Interventional Neuroradiology in the Treatment of CVT

Pharmacological Thrombectomy

Case Series

Vines and Davis [19] were the first to report on the use of urokinase in CVT, followed 10 years later by Di Rocco et al. [20], who successfully treated 5 patients with intravenous urokinase and heparin. In 1988, Scott et al. [21] reported on the first case of local fibrinolytic therapy in a young patient with an extensive superior sagittal sinus thrombosis. A local urokinase infusion was performed via a frontal burr hole and the patient who had initially been decerebrate made a good recovery despite the occurrence of a posttreatment hemorrhagic changes. About 30 cases of local urokinase infusion have been reported up to now, with doses ranging from 0.47 to 13.79 million units, delivered either through the internal jugular or femoral routes.

Barnwell et al. [22] reported on 3 patients, aged 51–71 years, having symptomatic dural sinus thrombosis with occlusion, who were treated with direct sinus perfusion with urokinase. All 3 patients had a dural arteriovenous fistula; 1 involving the inferior petrosal sinus and 2 involving the transverse sinus. All 3 patients were administered a transjugular direct infusion of urokinase. In 1 patient, a transfemoral venous approach was initially used but had to be discontinued because of an infection. The period of continuous infusion for thrombolysis ranged between 4 and 10 days. In 2 patients, the clinical signs and symptoms improved along with the angiographic evidence of clot lysis and dural sinus recanalization. Angiography showed that 1 patient had only a partial resolution of the torcular herophili and transverse sinus clot and no clinical improvement was observed.

The largest series to date has been that by Horowitz et al. [12] who treated 13 patients with extensive thrombosis of several sinuses: superior sagittal sinus (n = 12), lateral sinus (n = 12) and straight sinus (n = 4). Sinus patency and good recovery were obtained in 12 patients. There was no clinical worsening despite the presence of hemorrhagic infarct in 4 of these patients. Smith et al. [23] retrospectively reviewed 7 patients, aged 25–71 years, who presented symptomatic dural sinus thrombosis and failed to respond to medical therapy. Therefore, it was decided to treat the occluded sinuses with urokinase locally, with doses ranging from 20,000 to 150,000 U/h and a mean infusion time of

163 h (range 88–244 h). Patency of the affected dural sinus was achieved with anterograde flow in all patients. Six patients either improved neurologically or were healthy after thrombolysis; 1 patient requiring angioplasty. Another patient improved after the surgical repair of a residual dural arteriovenous fistula. Globally, the only complications observed were an infected femoral access site which resolved after antibiotic treatment and a hematuria which cleared up after discontinuing anticoagulants.

Wasay et al. [24] reviewed 40 consecutive patients with superior sagittal sinus thrombosis from 1981 to 1997, who had been treated with local urokinase (thrombolysis group) or systemic heparin anticoagulation (heparin group). The thrombolysis group (n = 20) received local urokinase into the superior sagittal sinus followed by systemic heparin anticoagulation. Both groups were similar for age, sex, baseline venous infarction and predisposing illnesses. Pretreatment neurological function was reported to be worse in the thrombolysis group (normal, n = 5; mild, n = 8; moderate, n = 4; severe, n = 3) than in the heparin group (normal, n = 8; mild, n = 8; moderate, n = 3; severe, n = 1; p = NS). Discharge neurological function was reported to be better in the thrombolysis group (normal, n = 16; mild, n = 3; moderate, n = 1; severe, n = 0) than in the heparin group (normal, n = 9; mild, n = 6; moderate, n = 5; severe, n = 0; p = 0.019). The rate of hemorrhagic complication was 10% (n = 2) in the thrombolysis group (subdural hematoma, retroperitoneal hemorrhage) and 0% in the heparin group (p = 0.49). Three of the heparin group patients developed CVT related complications such as: status epilepticus, hydrocephalus and refractory papilledema. There were no reported deaths in the two groups. Symptom duration in the thrombolysis group ranged from 1 day to 6 months, but all patients with chronic symptoms had previously either worsening or had developed new neurological symptoms or deficits. The length of hospital stay was similar in both groups.

Recombinant tissue plasminogen activator therapy (rtPA) has been used in combination with heparin because of its theoretical advantages which have demonstrated a capacity to decrease hemorrhagic risk. r-tPA is clot selective, has a short time life of 7–8 min, avoids plasminemia and produces the lowest level of fibrinogen degradation products [25–27].

Kim and Suh [26] published data on the treatment of 9 patients. Average duration of symptoms before treatment was 29 days (range: 7–112 days). Symptoms and signs reported in the study were: headache, seizure, lethargy/somnolence, hemiparesis, and papilledema. Pretreatment MR and CT brain scans were normal in 3 and showed minimal brain swelling and/or sulcal effacement in 5. Intracerebral hemorrhage (ICH) with venous infarct in the right parietal lobe was present in 1. Mean total dose of rtPA was 135 mg delivered over 20 h (range: 8–43 h), with concomitant intravenous heparin. Flow was re-established in all patients, including 1 who had had an involvement of both convexity and deep systems. No posttreatment brain hemorrhages were observed while clinical signs and symptoms, including neurologic deficits, seizures, and headaches, were treated successfully in all patients during the 3-month follow-up period. Two hemorrhagic complications were reported: groin bleeding requiring no treatment in one patient and intraperitoneal hemorrhage caused by hypofibrinogenemia requiring infusion of fresh-frozen plasma in another.

Frey et al. [25] reported on 12 patients with pretreatment symptoms lasting 1–40 days (e.g. headache, somnolence, focal deficits, seizures, and nausea and vomiting). Pretreatment MRI disclosed subtle hemorrhagic venous infarction in 4 patients, clear evidence of hemorrhagic infarction in 2, small parenchymal hemorrhage from recent pallidotomy in 1, and no focal lesions in 5 patients. Magnetic resonance venography and contrast venography identified thrombi in the superior sagittal sinuses of 3 patients; transverse/sigmoid sinuses in 2; superior sagittal sinus and both transverse/sigmoid sinuses in 1; superior sagittal sinus and one transverse/sigmoid sinus in 5; and superior sagittal sinus, transverse/sigmoid sinuses in 1, and straight sinus in 1. A loading dose of rtPA was instilled throughout the clot at 1 mg/cm, followed by continuous intrathrombus infusion at 1–2 mg/h and intravenous heparin was infused concomitantly. Flow was restored completely in 6 patients and partially in 3, with a mean rtPA dose of 46 mg (range, 23–128 mg) over a mean time of 29 h (range, 13–77 h). Symptoms improved in these latter 9 patients concomitantly with flow restoration. Flow could not be restored in 3 patients. In one of these, it was decided to stop treatment due to a decrease in the fibrinogen level to 118 mg/dl and only limited flow could be restored. Likewise, in the other 2 patients, hemorrhagic worsening occurred, and treatment was ceased after initial rtPA dosing. In one of these, the hematoma was evacuated.

This series by Frey et al. [25] is by far the largest to date, and taken together with the other reported series here [25] they provided data supporting the safety and efficacy of r-tPA in CVT. Complete flow restoration was achieved in most cases (6/12 in the Frey study [25] and 9/9 in the Kim and Suh series [26]) while there was a complete recovery in 5 out of 12 and 9 out of 9 cases, respectively. Moreover, the average flow restoration in both studies was reported to be rapid: 29 and 18 h, respectively. Although no such reliable data are available on the use heparin in CVT, it is an undeniable fact that complete recanalization with rtPA plus heparin is more effective than heparin alone. Equally, rtPA has been shown to be more effective than urokinase (an average of 71 h for 29 patients). However, it is noteworthy to report that recanalization had been obtained even in patients treated long after symptom onset, up to 16 weeks in 1 case [26], even though the correlation between flow restoration and clinical recovery was not complete.

Actually, 1 patient improved despite an absence of flow restoration, and 2 patients completely recovered even though incomplete flow restoration was observed in both. On the other hand, 1 patient had flow restoration but did not fully recover. Other flow parameters, such as collateral circulation, are thought to play a significant role in clinical recovery. This latter outcome measure has been proven through research as the most significant endpoint for the evaluation of treatment efficacy.

Regarding local rtPA, it carries an indisputable risk. In the Korean study [26], there were two reported complications: a minor bleeding at the femoral puncture site and a major intrapelvic hemorrhage requiring the administration of blood products. In the American study [25], 2 patients worsened because of increased intracerebral bleeding, which required surgery in one case.

Yamini et al. [28] described a patient with superior sagittal sinus thrombosis plus both transverse and straight sinuses and extension in the internal cerebral veins. This patient was treated with a local infusion of rt-PA into the superior sagittal sinus. The superior sagittal sinus was catheterized via a transfemoral route and then infused with 25 mg of rt-PA. No significant change in the severity of the thrombosis was observed and being so, the catheter was left in place and rt-PA was further infused at 1 mg/min for 19 h. At this point, an angiography was repeated which evidenced thrombosis resolution [28]. The authors sustained that a successfully completed lysis of the clot in the deep venous system can be achieved when infusion is performed directly inside the superior sagittal sinus [28]. Furthermore, the authors claimed that this result was due to the diffusion of rt-PA throughout the intracranial venous system or to the improved venous outflow caused by the clot lysis inside the superficial dural sinus [28].

Since 1971, more than 100 cases of CVT treated with urokinase or rt-PA have been reported on. We have brought together the main studies of CVT-related thrombolysis procedures found in literature up to now (table 1).

Randomized Controlled Trials

To date there have been no randomized controlled trials (RCTs) on thrombolytic therapy and CVT.

Mechanical Thrombectomy

Case Series

One of the limits of thrombolysis treatment for CVT is that it is most often complicated by hemorrhagic lesions. Thus, this fear that hemorrhagic stroke can deteriorate due to thrombolysis treatment leads to the development of improved

Table 1. Main studies of CVT-related thrombolysis procedures found in the literature (Wasay, modified)

First author	Patients	Agent	Pretreatment hemorrhage	Exacerbation of hemorrhagic component	NA	Outcome			Major complication
						good	poor	death	
Horowitz [12]	13	urokinase	4	0	1	11		1	retroperitoneal bleed (n = 1)
Frey [25]	12	tPA	7	2		9	3		none
Kim [26]	9	tPA	1	0		9			retroperitoneal bleed (n = 1)
Smith [23]	7	urokinase	N/A			7			none
Tsai [37]	5	urokinase	0			4	1		none
Kasner [38]	3	urokinase	3	0		3			none
Barnwell [22]	3	urokinase	N/A			2			none
Smith [23]	2	urokinase	1	0		3			none
Rael [39]	1	urokinase	1	0		1			none
Kermode [40]	1	streptokinase	0			1			none
Renowden [27]	1	tPA	0			1			none
Spearman [41]	2	urokinase	1	1		2	1		none
Crawford [42]	1	urokinase	N/A						N/A
Khoo [43]	1	urokinase	0			1			ICH
Gerszten [44]	1	urokinase	1	1		1			none
Griesemer [45]	1	urokinase	0			1			none
Eskridge [46]	1	urokinase	0			1			none
Manthous [47]	1	urokinase	0			1			none
Takami [48]	1	urokinase	0			1			none
D'Alise [49]	1	urokinase	0			1			none
Niwa [50]	1	tPA	0			1			none
Kuether [51]	1	urokinase	1	0		1			none

Smadja [52]	1	urokinase	0		1			hematuria (n = 1)
Satake [53]	1	urokinase	0	N/A	1			N/A
Manzione [54]	1	urokinase	0	0	1			none
Chow [55]	2	urokinase + reolysis	2	1	2			
Gurley [56]	2	urokinase	0	0	2			
Wasay [24]	20	urokinase	3	0	19	1	0	retroperitoneal bleed = 1; subdural hemorrhage = 1
Yamini [28]	1	tPA	NA		1			
Total	97				20	6	1	7

Outcome was assessed by the 4-point ordinal scale of neuroscores: 0 = normal; 1 = mild (able to ambulate and communicate); 2 = moderate (unable to ambulate, normal mentation); and 3 = severe (unable to ambulate, altered mentation).

mechanical techniques that lower the risk of bleeding. One of these devices is the rheolytic thrombectomy, which utilizes the Venturi effect which creates a negative pressure fragmenting and aspirating the cerebral venous thrombus. This pneumatic thrombectomy catheter was designed to alleviate acute vascular thrombosis; its catheter has both an inflow and outflow lumen. In fact, the inflow lumen carries normal saline under high pressure (approximately 9,000 psi) to the catheter nozzle at which point the flow reverses flow by 180°, and directs it back to the outflow lumen. By directing input flow into the area around the outflow lumen at a high speed (350–450 km/h), a negative pressure is created around the incoming flow vortex until the outflow lumen. The low-pressure area that is created by an adjacent high pressure is referred to as the Venturi effect. Three additional low-flow nozzles (25–40 km/h) from the input lumen are placed proximal to the high-speed nozzle. These three nozzles are perpendicularly directed to the catheter and create enough force to dislodge small portions of the thrombus and optimize the vortex at the outflow lumen [29]. The combination of these different pressures guarantees a successful removal of the thrombus from the artery or vein and draining into the outflow lumen.

The rheolytic thrombectomy catheter has been evaluated in in vitro studies and has shown to be minimally traumatic to vascular endothelium. Investigators have demonstrated that the rheolytic thrombectomy catheter can reanalyze saphrenous vein grafts and limb vessels that have been obstructed by diffused atherosclerosis and intraluminal thrombus [30]. The rheolytic thrombectomy catheter has also been used with success for angioscopic evaluations of coronary vein grafts. Opatowsky et al. [29], reported on the first ever case of rapid thrombectomy for extensive thrombus within the superior sagittal and transverse sinuses using a rheolytic catheter device. This patient was initially treated with a total of 750,000 U of urokinase infused over 90 min. During posttreatment, the patient's clinical status markedly worsened. Being so, the patient underwent a further angiographic assessment. Despite the first endovascular treatment, transvenous catheterization evidenced a complete rethrombosis of the dural sinuses. Faced with this clinical reality, even in the lack of clinical evidence, the decision was taken to perform a mechanical thrombectomy. With the patient under general anesthesia, a rheolytic thrombectomy catheter (AngioJet LF140; Possis Medical, Minneapolis, Minn., USA) was advanced over a 300-cm, 0.014-inch ACS Hi-Torque wire (Advanced Cardiovascular Systems, Temecula, Calif., USA). Buckling of the introducer catheter within the right side of the heart necessitated the introduction of a long 7F sheath (Cook Inc, Bloomington, Ind., USA) through which a 7F Brite Tip catheter (Cordis Corp, Miami, Fla., USA) was advanced. The thrombectomy catheter was then reintroduced coaxially and used to treat the entire length of the superior sagittal sinus as well as the bilateral transverse sinuses. This resulted in a markedly improved angiographic appearance of the superior sagittal sinus with minimal residual thrombus. The right transverse sinus showed slow anterograde flow. Infusion of 450,000 U of urokinase was then administered via a microcatheter throughout the sinus system. The resulting venous images were quite satisfactory. A posttreatment CT scan showed no evidence of complicating hemorrhage [29]. The same research group reported on a case series of 5 patients with dural sinus thrombosis who were all treated with a combination of pharmacological and mechanical thrombolysis using the 5-French AngioJet rheolytic catheter (Possis Medical) and balloon catheters. All 5 patients demonstrated immediate improvement which was confirmed on imaging studies or from neurological status. Three patients required more than one intervention, and all but one went on to improve after their final intervention. Two of the 5 patients continued to experience mild residual neurological deficits, whereas 2 patients completely recovered. The 5th patient had a delayed recurrence of thrombosis that required multiple interventions, leading to significant neurological deficits. Navigation of the dural sinuses was possible in all of the patients with a microcatheter and equally possible, to a variable degree, with a rheolytic catheter. Procedure complications included two pseudoaneurysms at the femoral puncture site [29].

A 34-year-old female nonsmoker on oral contraceptives with a middle-ear infection was treated by Scarrow et al. [31] for right transverse and sigmoid sinus thromboses. A microcatheter (Tracker 18 MX, Target Therapeutics, Freemont, Calif., USA) with its wire was placed into the thrombus. After much difficulty in getting it through the length of the thrombus, a patent torcula was reached. At this point, the microcatheter and base catheters were substituted for a 7F guide catheter and a rheolytic thrombectomy catheter (CF105 AngioJet, POSSIS Medical, Inc., Minneapolis, Minn., USA). The exchange wire was positioned across the torcula in the opposite sigmoid sinus during the exchange. The rheolytic thrombectomy catheter easily followed the 0.014-inch guide wire even through the clot which had previously been extremely resistant. The rheolytic thrombectomy catheter was then activated and slowly withdrawn at 1–2 mm/s. A retrograde venogram obtained via the base catheter showed some patency within 5 min. Several more passes were made with the thrombectomy catheter, advancing it back to the torcula and withdrawing it again. The final venogram (obtained 17 min from mechanical disruption) showed excellent flow despite residual thrombus. Thrombolytic infusion was not performed owing to the good angiographic result and observed rapid clinical improvement.

Chahlavi et al. [32] presented two cases of direct dural sinus thrombosis thrombectomy performed using a rheolytic catheter via a transcranial route. These two patients had been neurologically deteriorating and the attempted transfemoral catheter approach was unsuccessful. Being so, a mechanical thrombectomy passing through a burr hole over the dural sinus (transcranial approach) was performed. With this approach, it was possible to bypass the tortuous intracranial vascular anatomy with the large and rheolytic catheter [32].

Recently, Kirsch et al. [33] has published a retrospective review of a prospective database. Here, the authors described 4 patients ranging in age from 28 to 67 years (3 female, 1 male) with CVT and rapidly deteriorating levels of consciousness who underwent transfemoral intravenous rheolytic thrombectomy utilizing AngioJet XMI and/or Xpeedior catheters (Possis Medical). All 4 patients had successful mechanical thrombectomy as evidenced by their blood flow restorations. A normalization of angiographic transit time after thrombectomy was evidenced in 3 of the 4 patients who also had a rapid neurological improvement. The 4th patient died during the periprocedural period. No procedural complications were reported in any of the patients.

Randomized Controlled Trials

To date, there have been no randomized controlled trials carried out on mechanical thrombectomy in CVT.

Combinations of Pharmacological and Mechanical Treatments

Case Series

Dowd et al. [34] described the application of a rheolytic thrombectomy system for the treatment of symptomatic dural sinus thrombosis in a 54-year-old female with somnolence and left-sided weakness. A diagnosis of bilateral transverse and superior sagittal sinus thrombosis was made and thus the patient was treated with anticoagulant therapy. Eight days after presentation, following an initial period of improvement, the patient entered into coma and the left-side weakness worsened into hemiplegia. After excluding intracerebral hemorrhage by MRI, angiography and transfemoral venous thrombolysis with a hydrodynamic thrombectomy catheter were performed. This was proceeded by intrasinus urokinase thrombolytic therapy for 48 h, resulting in a complete clot thrombolysis leading to an almost complete neurologic recovery. Six months after treatment, the patient had mild cognitive impairment and no focal neurologic deficits [34]. Curtin et al. [35] described a case of a 28-year-old female with bilateral anterior parietal lobe cortical hemorrhages associated with thrombosis of the superior sagittal sinus, both transverse and sigmoid sinuses, and multiple cortical veins draining into the sagittal sinus. An 8F shuttle (Cook, Bloomington, Ind., USA) 90-cm sheath was inserted through the right femoral vein directing the catheter tip slightly below the right jugular bulb. A 135-cm Turbo Tracker 18 catheter (Boston Scientific, Natick, Mass., USA) and a 150-cm 0.018-inch Terumo gold Glidewire were navigated into the superior sagittal sinus; gentle contrast injection showed

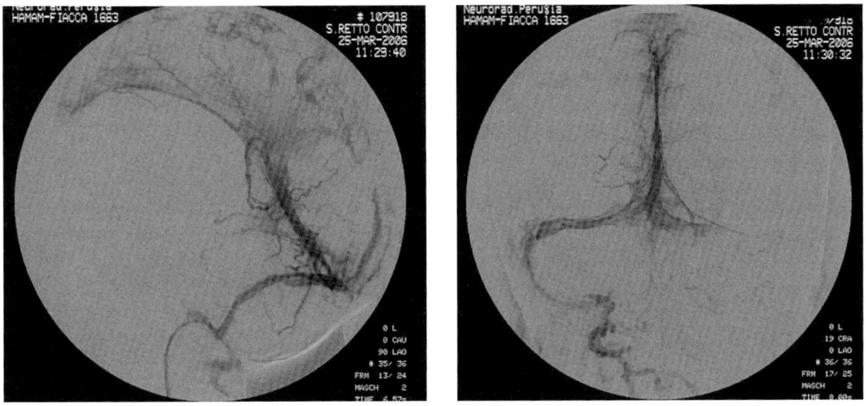

a b

Fig. 1. ***a*** Thrombosis of the straight sinus, sinus rectus, sinus transversus with cerebral hypertension. ***b*** Delayed visualization of the right jugularis vein.

minimal venous outflow running anteriorly (retrograde to normal flow direction) and extensive clot filling the superior sagittal sinus. A 135-cm 4F AngioJet catheter (Possis Medical) was directed over a 0.14-inch ACS Hi-Torque Extrasport 300-cm exchange wire (Advanced Cardiovascular Systems) into the superior sagittal sinus. With the Possis rheolytic thrombectomy system engaged, the AngioJet catheter was withdrawn towards the right jugular bulb and then returned to the superior sagittal sinus. Venography performed via the AngioJet catheter port showed improved patency of the superior sagittal and right transverse sinuses, with slow antegrade flow, although considerable clotting remained. The Tracker 18 catheter and 0.18-inch gold Glidewire were used to cross the midline and to catheterize the thrombosed left transverse and sigmoid sinuses. The 4F AngioJet catheter was positioned within the left sigmoid sinus near the left jugular bulb over the exchange wire, then withdrawn until the midline, and then once again advanced performing rheolytic thrombectomy on both passes. A 120-cm, 5 × 20 mm Slalom angioplasty balloon (Cordis, Miami Lakes, Fla., USA) was inflated to 3–4 atm in the mid to distal right transverse sinus, the area in which most of the focal thrombotic stenosis still remained. There was no attempt to use a balloon such as a 'Fogarty', to proximally remove the thrombus. A control venography via the Tracker catheter in the superior sagittal sinus showed slow antegrade flow and considerable thrombus still present within the superior sagittal sinus and both transverse and both sigmoid sinuses. Continuous infusion thrombolytic therapy was initiated with the Tracker tip inside the superior sagittal sinus midportion at a velocity of 0.3 mg/h of r-TPA.

An example is given of thrombosis of the straight sinus, sinus rectus, sinus transversus with cerebral hypertension (fig. 1) treated with thrombectomy

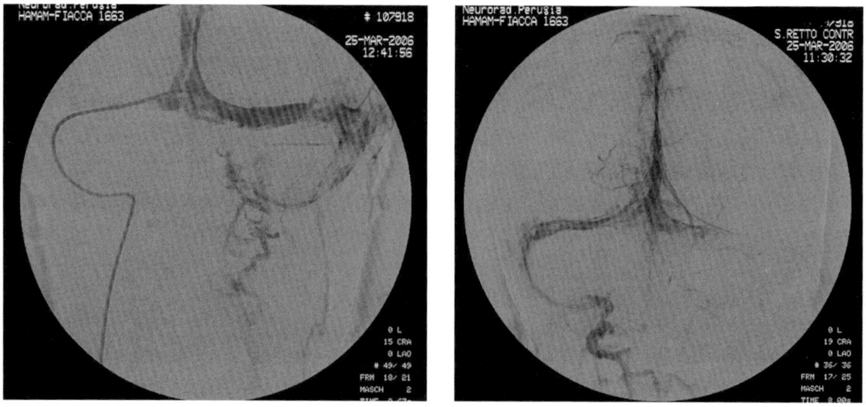

a *b*

Fig. 2. Thrombectomy followed by urokinase administration (1,200,000 UI). Catheterization of the sinus rectus to the vein of Galen, sinus sagittalis and torcula (***a***) and mechanical thromboaspiration (***b***).

followed by urokinase administration (1,200,000 UI) with catheterization of the sinus rectus to the vein of Galen, sinus sagittalis and torcula (fig. 2).

Randomized Controlled Trials

Currently there are no data on RCTs regarding the combinations of mechanical and pharmacological thrombectomy and CVT.

Efficacy and Safety of Interventional Neuroradiology

The interventional neuroradiology data presented in this chapter appear very promising for their efficacy and feasibility for patients with CVT.

Even though more and more physicians are choosing to treat CVT patients with local endovascular urokinase or rtPA, the benefit to risk ratio of these treatments is still unknown. From what has been reported in the literature, local thrombolysis is believed to better restore venous blood flow than heparin alone. This is so, even in the absence of clear evidence from randomized trials that clinical outcome is superior. Furthermore, in theory, hemorrhagic risk is higher in thrombolysis compared to heparin, especially when a pretreatment hemorrhage is already present.

Thrombolysis is also used when the patient's condition worsens despite heparin and symptomatic treatment. The most frequently described cause of worsening is inadequate anticoagulation. Clinical deterioration due to thrombosis progression in properly anticoagulated patients is rarely observed. When it is observed, a thrombolytic treatment should be considered as a valid option [36].

To understand the true efficacy of thrombolytic treatment, publication selection bias must be taken into account. The authors here hold that the best way to fully understand the benefits related to interventional neuroradiological treatment would be to design a randomized trial comparing this treatment with heparin for CVT.

Proposals for the Use of Interventional Neuroradiology

Are There Cases Where Interventional Neuroradiology Can Be Used without RCTs?

In the absence of RCTs showing any benefit of interventional radiology over intravenous heparin therapy, it cannot be recommended to use interventional radiological techniques in CVT patients who have a good chance to survive without sequelae, i.e. those with normal consciousness, no cerebral hemorrhage or infarct, no sign of encephalopathy, isolated intracranial hypertension or headache, no focal deficit [3–9, 11, 13–18]. Those who seem to be the most appropriate candidates for interventional radiology are therefore those who worsen despite heparin or are in a too poor status to wait for the effect of heparin. Those patients are those who (a) have predictors of poor outcome such as coma (not related to seizures), or occlusions of several sinuses or veins, and (b) those who worsen despite a properly administered and monitored anticoagulation by heparin, in the absence of other explanation (especially seizures).

Need for a Clinical Randomized Trial

The question whether 1st line interventional radiology is more effective or safer than heparin therapy even in patients who can be treated by heparin can only be answered by RCTs. The is no reason to recommend interventional radiology in these patients who are likely to have a good outcome unless proven superior in a trial.

Acknowledgment

The authors are grateful to Dr. Mohammed Hamam and Andrea Fiacca for the excellent angiographic scans.

References

1 Burt RL, Donnelly JF, Whitener DL: Cerebral venous thrombosis in the puerperium; report of two cases with necropsy findings. Am J Obstet Gynecol 1951;62:639–643.
2 Barnett HJ, Hyland HH: Noninfective intracranial venous thrombosis. Brain 1953;76:36–49.
3 Breteau G, Mounier-Vehier F, Godefroy O, Gauvrit JY, Mackowiak-Cordoliani MA, Girot M, Bertheloot D, Henon H, Lucas C, Leclerc X, Fourrier F, Pruvo JP, Leys D: Cerebral venous thrombosis 3-year clinical outcome in 55 consecutive patients. J Neurol 2003;250:29–35.
4 Ferro JM, Canhao P, Stam J, Bousser MG, Barinagarrementeria F: Prognosis of cerebral vein and dural sinus thrombosis: results of the International Study on Cerebral Vein and Dural Sinus Thrombosis (ISCVT). Stroke 2004;35:664–670.
5 Rondepierre P, Hamon M, Leys D, Leclerc X, Mounier-Vehier F, Godefroy O, Janssens E, Pruvo JP: Thromboses veineuses cérébrales: étude de l'évolution. Rev Neurol (Paris) 1995;151: 100–104.
6 Bousser MG: Cerebral venous thrombosis: diagnosis and management. J Neurol 2000;247:252–258.
7 Biousse V, Ameri A, Bousser MG: Isolated intracranial hypertension as the only sign of cerebral venous thrombosis. Neurology 1999;53:1537–1542.
8 Biousse V, Tong F, Newman NJ: Cerebral venous thrombosis. Curr Treat Options Neurol 2003;5:409–420.
9 Bousser MG, Chiras J, Bories J, Castaigne P: Cerebral venous thrombosis – a review of 38 cases. Stroke 1985;16:199–213.
10 Einhaupl KM, Villringer A, Meister W, Mehraein S, Garner C, Pellkofer M, Haberl RL, Pfister HW, Schmiedek P: Heparin treatment in sinus venous thrombosis. Lancet 1991;338:597–600.
11 Girot M, Ferro JM, Canhao P, Stam J, Bousser MG, Barinagarrementeria F, Leys D: Predictors of outcome in patients with cerebral venous thrombosis and intracerebral hemorrhage. Stroke 2007;38:337–342.
12 Horowitz M, Purdy P, Unwin H, Carstens G 3rd, Greenlee R, Hise J, Kopitnik T, Batjer H, Rollins N, Samson D: Treatment of dural sinus thrombosis using selective catheterization and urokinase. Ann Neurol 1995;38:58–67.
13 Bienfait HP, Stam J, Lensing AW, van Hilten JJ: Trombose van de cerebrale venen en sinussen bij 62 patienten. Ned Tijdschr Geneeskd 1995;139:1286–1291.
14 de Bruijn SF, de Haan RJ, Stam J; for The Cerebral Venous Sinus Thrombosis Study Group: Clinical features and prognostic factors of cerebral venous sinus thrombosis in a prospective series of 59 patients. J Neurol Neurosurg Psychiatry 2001;70:105–108.
15 Ferro JM, Correia M, Pontes C, Baptista MV, Pita F: Cerebral vein and dural sinus thrombosis in Portugal: 1980–1998. Cerebrovasc Dis 2001;11:177–182.
16 Mehraein S, Schmidtke K, Villringer A, Valdueza JM, Masuhr F: Heparin treatment in cerebral sinus and venous thrombosis: patients at risk of fatal outcome. Cerebrovasc Dis 2003;15: 17–21.
17 Bell DA, Davis WL, Osborn AG, Harnsberger HR: Bithalamic hyperintensity on T_2-weighted MR: vascular causes and evaluation with MR angiography. AJNR Am J Neuroradiol 1994;15:893–899.
18 Magni C, Mocaer J, Yapo P, Bibi R, Cazeneuve N, Ferquel C, Agnard P, Friocourt P: Les thromboses veineuses cérébrales profondes. J Neuroradiol 1998;25:116–122.
19 Vines FS, Davis DO: Clinical-radiological correlation in cerebral venous occlusive disease. Radiology 1971;98:9–22.
20 Di Rocco C, Iannelli A, Leone G, Moschini M, Valori VM: Heparin-urokinase treatment in aseptic dural sinus thrombosis. Arch Neurol 1981;38:431–435.
21 Scott JA, Pascuzzi RM, Hall PV, Becker GJ: Treatment of dural sinus thrombosis with local urokinase infusion. Case report. J Neurosurg 1988;68:284–287.
22 Barnwell SL, Higashida RT, Halbach VV, Dowd CF, Hieshima GB: Direct endovascular thrombolytic therapy for dural sinus thrombosis. Neurosurgery 1991;28:135–142.
23 Smith TP, Higashida RT, Barnwell SL, Halbach VV, Dowd CF, Fraser KW, Teitelbaum GP, Hieshima GB: Treatment of dural sinus thrombosis by urokinase infusion. AJNR Am J Neuroradiol 1994;15:801–807.

24 Wasay M, Bakshi R, Kojan S, Bobustuc G, Dubey N, Unwin DH: Nonrandomized comparison of local urokinase thrombolysis versus systemic heparin anticoagulation for superior sagittal sinus thrombosis. Stroke 2001;32:2310–2317.
25 Frey JL, Muro GJ, McDougall CG, Dean BL, Jahnke HK: Cerebral venous thrombosis: combined intrathrombus rtPA and intravenous heparin. Stroke 1999;30:489–494.
26 Kim SY, Suh JH: Direct endovascular thrombolytic therapy for dural sinus thrombosis: infusion of alteplase. AJNR Am J Neuroradiol 1997;18:639–645.
27 Renowden SA, Oxbury J, Molyneux AJ: Case report: venous sinus thrombosis: the use of thrombolysis. Clin Radiol 1997;52:396–399.
28 Yamini B, Loch Macdonald R, Rosenblum J: Treatment of deep cerebral venous thrombosis by local infusion of tissue plasminogen activator. Surg Neurol 2001;55:340–346.
29 Opatowsky MJ, Morris PP, Regan JD, Mewborne JD, Wilson JA: Rapid thrombectomy of superior sagittal sinus and transverse sinus thrombosis with a rheolytic catheter device. AJNR Am J Neuroradiol 1999;20:414–417.
30 Silva JA, Ramee SR, Collins TJ, Jenkins JS, Lansky AJ, Ansel GM, Dolmatch BL, Glickman MH, Stainken B, Ramee E, White CJ: Rheolytic thrombectomy in the treatment of acute limb-threatening ischemia: immediate results and six-month follow-up of the multicenter AngioJet registry. Possis Peripheral AngioJet Study AngioJet Investigators. Cathet Cardiovasc Diagn 1998;45:386–393.
31 Scarrow AM, Williams RL, Jungreis CA, Yonas H, Scarrow MR: Removal of a thrombus from the sigmoid and transverse sinuses with a rheolytic thrombectomy catheter. AJNR Am J Neuroradiol 1999;20:1467–1469.
32 Chahlavi A, Steinmetz MP, Masaryk TJ, Rasmussen PA: A transcranial approach for direct mechanical thrombectomy of dural sinus thrombosis. Report of two cases. J Neurosurg 2004;101: 347–351.
33 Kirsch J, Rasmussen PA, Masaryk TJ, Perl J 2nd, Fiorella D: Adjunctive rheolytic thrombectomy for central venous sinus thrombosis: technical case report. Neurosurgery 2007;60:E577–578; discussion E578.
34 Dowd CF, Malek AM, Phatouros CC, Hemphill JC 3rd: Application of a rheolytic thrombectomy device in the treatment of dural sinus thrombosis: a new technique. AJNR Am J Neuroradiol 1999;20:568–570.
35 Curtin KR, Shaibani A, Resnick SA, Russell EJ, Simuni T: Rheolytic catheter thrombectomy, balloon angioplasty, and direct recombinant tissue plasminogen activator thrombolysis of dural sinus thrombosis with preexisting hemorrhagic infarctions. AJNR Am J Neuroradiol 2004;25: 1807–1811.
36 Bousser MG: Cerebral venous thrombosis: nothing, heparin, or local thrombolysis? Stroke 1999;30:481–483.
37 Tsai FY, Higashida RT, Matovich V, Alfieri K: Acute thrombosis of the intracranial dural sinus: direct thrombolytic treatment. AJNR Am J Neuroradiol 1992;13:1137–1141.
38 Kasner S, Gurian J, Grotta J: Urokinase treatment of sagittal sinus thrombosis with venous hemorrhagic infarctions. J Stroke Cerebrovasc Dis 1998;7:421–425.
39 Rael JR, Orrison WW Jr, Baldwin N, Sell J: Direct thrombolysis of superior sagittal sinus thrombosis with coexisting intracranial hemorrhage. AJNR Am J Neuroradiol 1997;18: 1238–1242.
40 Kermode AG, Ives FJ, Taylor B, Davis SJ, Carroll WM: Progressive dural venous sinus thrombosis treated with local streptokinase infusion. J Neurol Neurosurg Psychiatry 1995;58:107–108.
41 Spearman MP, Jungreis CA, Wehner JJ, Gerszten PC, Welch WC: Endovascular thrombolysis in deep cerebral venous thrombosis. AJNR Am J Neuroradiol 1997;18:502–506.
42 Crawford SC, Digre KB, Palmer CA, Bell DA, Osborn AG: Thrombosis of the deep venous drainage of the brain in adults. Analysis of seven cases with review of the literature. Arch Neurol 1995;52:1101–1108.
43 Khoo KB, Long FL, Tuck RR, Allen RJ, Tymms KE: Cerebral venous sinus thrombosis associated with the primary antiphospholipid syndrome. Resolution with local thrombolytic therapy. Med J Aust 1995;162:30–32.
44 Gerszten PC, Welch WC, Spearman MP, Jungreis CA, Redner RL: Isolated deep cerebral venous thrombosis treated by direct endovascular thrombolysis. Surg Neurol 1997;48:261–266.

45 Griesemer DA, Theodorou AA, Berg RA, Spera TD: Local fibrinolysis in cerebral venous thrombosis. Pediatr Neurol 1994;10:78–80.
46 Eskridge JM, Wessbecher FW: Thrombolysis for superior sagittal sinus thrombosis. J Vasc Interv Radiol 1991;2:89–93; discussion 93–84.
47 Manthous CA, Chen H: Case report: treatment of superior sagittal sinus thrombosis with urokinase. Conn Med 1992;56:529–530.
48 Takami T, Suzuki T, Tokuno H, Egashira M, Tsuyuguchi N, Komiyama M, Hakuba A: A case report of dural sinus thrombosis: direct thrombolytic therapy using endovascular surgery (in Japanese). No Shinkei Geka 1995;23:321–325.
49 D'Alise MD, Fichtel F, Horowitz M: Sagittal sinus thrombosis following minor head injury treated with continuous urokinase infusion. Surg Neurol 1998;49:430–435.
50 Niwa J, Ohyama H, Matumura S, Maeda Y, Shimizu T: Treatment of acute superior sagittal sinus thrombosis by t-PA infusion via venography – direct thrombolytic therapy in the acute phase. Surg Neurol 1998;49:425–429.
51 Kuether TA, O'Neill O, Nesbit GM, Barnwell SL: Endovascular treatment of traumatic dural sinus thrombosis: case report. Neurosurgery 1998;42:1163–1166; discussion 1166–1167.
52 Smadja D, Raynaud M, Mehdaoui H, Poey C, Drault JN, Ridarch A, Tixier F, Vernant JC, Mas JL: Thrombose veineuse cérébrale étendue résistante a l'héparine: fibrinolyse locale par urokinase. Rev Neurol (Paris) 1997;153:271–274.
53 Satake R, Arakawa S, Hashimoto M, Minamide H, Takamori M: Successful direct thrombolysis in a patient with extensive dural sinus thrombosis induced by danazol (in Japanese). Rinsho Shinkeigaku 1997;37:309–313.
54 Ouriel K, Shortell CK, DeWeese JA, Green RM, Francis CW, Azodo MV, Gutierrez OH, Manzione JV, Cox C, Marder VJ: A comparison of thrombolytic therapy with operative revascularization in the initial treatment of acute peripheral arterial ischemia. J Vasc Surg 1994;19:1021–1030.
55 Chow K, Gobin YP, Saver J, Kidwell C, Dong P, Vinuela F: Endovascular treatment of dural sinus thrombosis with rheolytic thrombectomy and intra-arterial thrombolysis. Stroke 2000;31: 1420–1425.
56 Gurley MB, King TS, Tsai FY: Sigmoid sinus thrombosis associated with internal jugular venous occlusion: direct thrombolytic treatment. J Endovasc Surg 1996;3:306–314.

Valeria Caso, MD, PhD
Stroke Unit and Division of Cardiovascular Medicine
Department of Internal Medicine, University of Perugia
Santa Maria della Misericordia Hospital
Via Dottori, Sant' Andrea delle Fratte, IT–06126 Perugia (Italy)
Tel./Fax +39 755 784 309, E-Mail stroke_unit@med.unipg.it

Caso V, Agnelli G, Paciaroni M (eds): Handbook on Cerebral Venous Thrombosis.
Front Neurol Neurosci. Basel, Karger, 2008, vol 23, pp 161–171

Complications of Cerebral Vein and Sinus Thrombosis

José M. Ferro, P. Canhão

Department of Neurology, Hospital de Santa Maria, Lisbon, Portugal

Abstract

Thrombosis of the dural sinus and encephalic veins (CVT) is an infrequent condition accounting for less than 1% of all strokes. Several recent prospective series, in particular the large International Study on Cerebral Vein and Dural Sinus Thrombosis cohort, definitely have shown a more benign prognosis compared with that of arterial strokes: CVT has an acute case fatality of less than 5%, and almost 80% of patients recover without sequelae. However, patients surviving the acute phase of CVT are at risk of a number of complications such as recurrence of any thrombotic events in about 7%, recurrence of CVT in about 2–12%, seizures in 5 to 32%, visual loss due to optic atrophy in percentages that range from less than 1 to 5%, presence of dural fistula (there are no data available about exact frequency) and neuropsychological and neuropsychiatric sequelae characterized by aphasia, abulia and depression. However, there is only little information on the long-term neuropsychological outcome. Studies investigating professional status, cognitive performance, depressive symptoms and quality of life evidenced depression and anxiety in 2/3 of CVT patients despite an apparent good recovery in 87% of these patients. Thus, patients should be encouraged to return to previous occupations and hobbies and reassured about the very low risk of recurrence.

Copyright © 2008 S. Karger AG, Basel

Complications of Cerebral Venous Thrombosis

Thrombosis of the dural sinus and encephalic veins (CVT) is an infrequent condition accounting for less than 1% of all strokes. It can occur at any age, and predominantly afflicts females and younger patients compared with other types of strokes [1].

Several recent prospective series, in particular the large International Study on Cerebral Vein and Dural Sinus Thrombosis (ISCVT) cohort [2–7], have definitely shown a more benign prognosis compared with that of arterial strokes:

Table 1. Frequency of thrombotic recurrent events after dural sinus thrombosis (CVT)

Study	Patients with follow-up	Length of follow-up	CVT	Other thrombotic events
Prospective				
ISCVT [2]	597	median 16 months mean 18.6 ± 11 months	14 (2.3)	27 (4.5)
VENOPORT[1] [5]	84	median 12 months mean 12 ± 7 months	0	5 (6)
Breteau et al. [6]	48	median 36 (12–60) months	0	3 (5.5)
Baumgartner et al. [10]	33	12 months	0	0
Rondepierre et al. [3]	18	6–30 months	0	1 (5.5)
Retrospective				
Gosk-Bierska et al. [9]	154	mean 36 ± 47 months	10 (6.5)	11 (7)
Preter et al. [8]	77	median 63 months mean 77.8 months	9 (11.7)	11 (14.3)
Masuhr et al. [11]	NK	10 years	5 (6)	NK
Maqueda and Thijs [12]	54	median 2.4 years mean 3.5 years	1 (1.9)	8 (14.8)

NK = Not known. Figures in parentheses indicate percentages.
[1]Prospective part of the study.

CVT has an acute case fatality of less than 5%, and almost 80% of patients recover without sequelae. Despite the overall favorable prognosis, patients surviving the acute phase of CVT are at risk of a number of complications.

Recurrence of Thrombotic Events

Patients suffering a CVT are likely to be at increased risk of having further thrombotic events. Venous thrombosis may recur in cerebral veins and dural sinus or may arise in different sites of the body. These complications were addressed in a few prospective studies collecting patients with CVT (table 1). Overall, during the follow-up about 7% of patients have any types of recurrent thrombosis [2, 5]. The risk may be increased in patients with a prothrombotic condition and the majority of recurrent events appear to occur during the 1st year after CVT [8, 9].

Recurrence of Cerebral Venous Thrombosis

The actual risk of CVT recurrence is very low. A few patients develop new signs or symptoms during the follow-up of CVT. To be sure that those symptoms are due to recurrent CVT, it has to be shown that new filling defects in veins or dural sinus observed on MRI/MRA were not evident in previous studies. For this purpose, it is crucial to have an MRI/MRA performed some months after the acute CVT phase, when recanalization has already occurred [10].

In the ISCVT study [2], recurrent sinus thrombosis was documented in 14 patients (2.3%), and none was reported in several prospective series [3, 6, 10] (table 1).

The frequency of CVT recurrence in retrospective studies varied from 2 to 12% [8, 9, 11, 12] (table 1). Gosk-Bierska et al. [9] described an even rate of recurrent CVT of 2.2/100 patient-years.

Influence of Recanalization on CVT Recurrence

Although is possible that incomplete or nonrecanalization of sinus after CVT could be a factor predisposing to CVT recurrence, the role of recanalization in further thrombotic events is unknown. Few studies analyzed dural sinus or venous recanalization after CVT [7, 10, 13–15], either to assess the time when recanalization of the dural sinus occurs after CVT [10], or the influence of sinus recanalization on the outcome of CVT [13]. Data on recurrent CVT were not reported in other studies addressing the topic of recanalization [14, 15].

Recurrence of Other Thrombotic Events

The frequency of thrombotic events other than CVT was reported in prospective studies (table 1). In the ISCVT [2], 4.5% of patients had recurrent thrombosis, more frequently in the peripheral venous system (limb or pelvic veins in 16 patients, pulmonary embolism in 3 patients) than in the arterial system (8 patients). In the prospective series of the VENOPORT study [5], recurrent thrombosis was also more frequent in veins (2 deep venous thrombosis, 1 pulmonary embolism).

Data from retrospective studies indicate a frequency between 7 and 14.8% of thrombotic events involving venous system (deep venous system, retinal vein, pulmonary thromboembolism, mesenteric vein) more often than arterial system [8, 9, 12]. Gosk-Bierska et al. [9] series estimated an event rate of recurrent events of 2.8/100 patient-years.

Due to the risk of thrombosis recurrence, it is recommended to continue oral anticoagulation after the acute phase for 6–12 months. The optimal duration of anticoagulation is unknown, and should be based on individual hereditary and precipitating factors. Long-term treatment should be considered for patients with a severe thrombophilia with high risk of recurrence, such as antithrombin deficiency, homozygous factor V Leiden mutation, or two or more thrombophilic conditions [16]. Indefinite anticoagulation is also considered in patients with two or more episodes of idiopathic documented extracerebral thrombosis [17].

Headache

Headache is the most frequent symptom in CVT, occurring isolated or with other symptoms or signs and reported in more than 80% of the patients [2].

Headache is also one of the most common complaints during the follow-up of CVT patients distressing about half of the patients [5, 6]. More frequently headache is benign, of migraine or tension type. In the Lille study, 53% of patients had residual headache, 29% fulfilled criteria for migraine and 27% were of tension type. In the VENOPORT, 55% of patients reported headaches during the follow-up, being mild to moderate in 45%.

Nevertheless, in some cases headache is very severe or prolonged. Severe headaches requiring bed rest or hospital admission were reported in 14% of patients in the ISCVT [2] and 11% in the VENOPORT [5]. Sometimes, it is mandatory to exclude recurrent CVT, by MRI/MRA. Occasionally MRV may depict stenosis of a previously occluded sinus but its clinical significance is still unclear.

The frequency or type of headaches during the follow-up may differ according to the initial clinical presentation syndrome of CVT. In the ISCVT study, patients with the isolated intracranial hypertension syndrome had more frequently severe headache during the follow-up compared with patients with other presentation syndromes (21 vs. 13%, $p = 0.019$) [18]. In a series of 17 patients presenting with headache as the only neurological sign of CVT, several patients had headaches at 3 months: migraine attacks similar to previous ones (4), tension type (2), and new onset of migraine with aura (2) [19].

In summary, the majority of headaches after CVT are benign. MRI/MRA is necessary in some cases to exclude the rare case of recurrent CVT. If headache persists and MRI is normal, a lumbar puncture may be needed to exclude elevated intracranial pressure (fig. 1). Repeated lumbar punctures, a lumbar-peritoneal shunt or stenting of a sinus stenosis are possible therapeutic options for persistent intracranial hypertension.

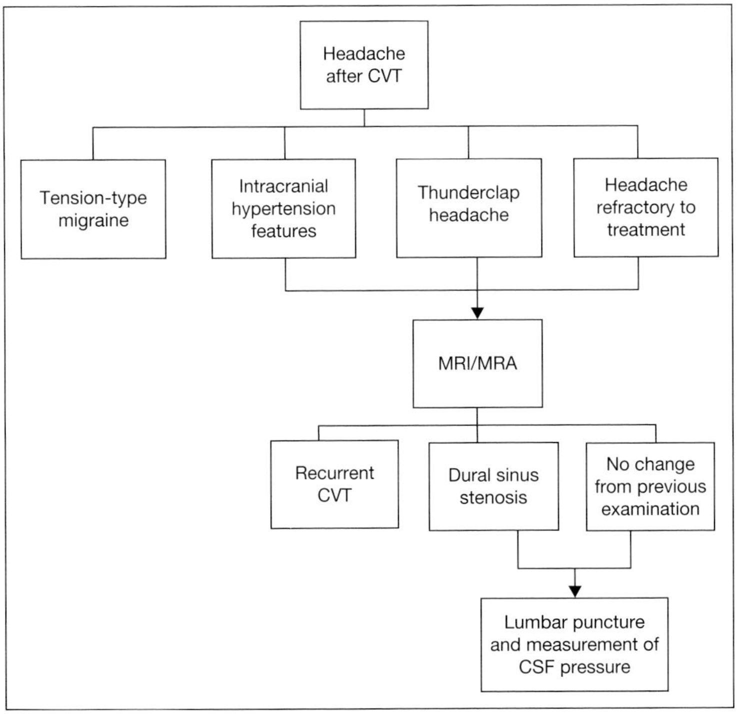

Fig. 1. Clinical assessment of headaches occurring after CVT.

Seizures

Focal or generalized poststroke seizures can be divided into early or remote [20]. The most used criteria for subdividing symptomatic seizures in CVT is considering remote seizures – those occurring [21, 22] more than 2 weeks after the confirmation of CVT diagnosis.

In a published case series, the percent of patients experiencing remote seizures ranged from 5 to 32%. In the series by Preter et al. [8], all remote seizures occurred in the 1st year of follow-up and were seen only in patients with seizures in the acute phase or with focal deficits. In the VENOPORT study [21], remote seizures occurred in 9.5% of the patients. Half of these patients had multiple seizures. Remote seizures were more frequent if the patient had seizures in the acute phase or had a hemorrhagic parenchymal lesion. All seizures occurred in the 1st year of follow-up. In ISCVT [2], 67 patients (10.7%) experienced remote seizures: 36 until the 6th month of follow-up, 55 until the 1 year, and 66 until the 2nd year. Risk factors for remote seizures were hemorrhagic lesion on admission CT/MR (HR = 2.62), early seizure (at presentation or <15 days after the diagnosis of CVT; HR = 2.42) and paresis (HR = 2.22). Twenty-nine patients (4.6%) had post-CVT epilepsy (more than one remote seizure). Post-CVT epilepsy was also associated with hemorrhagic lesion on admission CT/MR (OR = 6.76), early seizure (OR = 3.99) and paresis (OR = 2.75) [23].

The EFNS guidelines indicate as good practice points that prophylactic antiepileptic drugs (AEDs) may be a therapeutical option in patients with focal neurological deficits and focal parenchymal lesion on admission CT/MR [16].

The new information provided by the analysis of the ISCVT cohort [22, 23] enables a refinement of EFNS current recommendations. We recommend starting AEDs in any patient that presents with seizure or suffers an early or remote seizure. This indication is stronger in patients with supratentorial lesions, in particular if hemorrhagic. In addition, it is an acceptable option to prescribe AEDs for patients with a supratentorial hemorrhagic lesion or a motor defect but no seizure.

The optimal duration of AED treatment is unknown, but in general it is considered to be at least 1 year. General recommendations for the selection and withdrawal of AEDs can be used as options.

Visual Loss

Visual loss is not a frequent symptom in the acute phase of CVT, although as much as 30% of patients may have papilledema [2]. Severe papilledema can cause transient visual impairments, and if prolonged and left untreated optic atrophy and even blindness may ensue. Visual loss is often insidious, with progressive constriction of the visual fields and relative sparing of central visual acuity.

As many as 42 (6.7%) patients had visual complaints during the follow-up in the ISCVT study [2], most often subjective and not quantified by optometric or campimetric evaluation. Only 4 (<1%), had severe visual loss. In the prospective series of the VENOPORT [5] study, 7 patients (8%) had decreased visual acuity, severe in 1 patient (1%). This complication was also rare in the study by Preter et al. [8], where 2 patients (2.6%) were left with blindness due to optic atrophy. In the Lille study, 3 patients (5.5%) had visual field defects and 2 (3.6%) had a decreased visual acuity due to optic nerve atrophy [6]. Biousse et al. [24] systematically examined 59 out of 160 CVT consecutive patients with the isolated intracranial hypertension syndrome: 3 (5%) developed optic atrophy with severe visual loss.

Although a rare complication, visual loss should be investigated, actively prevented and treated. Patients with papilledema or visual complaints should have a complete study, including visual acuity and formal visual field testing. Increased intracranial pressure must be rapidly ruled out and treated. If vision continues to deteriorate despite acetazolamide and repeated lumbar punctures, a surgical treatment should be considered such as lumboperitoneal shunt or optic nerve sheath fenestration [16].

Dural Arteriovenous Fistula

Thrombosis of the cavernous, lateral or sagittal sinus can later induce a dural arteriovenous fistula [25]. A pial fistula can also follow a cortical vein thrombosis [26]. The relationship between the two entities is rather complex because: (1) dural fistulae can be a late complication of persistent dural sinus occlusion with increased venous pressure, (2) the fistula can close and cure if the sinus recanalizes, (3) a pre-existing fistula can be the underlying cause of CVT.

The exact frequency of dural fistula after CVT is not known, because there are no cohort studies with long-term angiographic investigation. Only 1 patient out of 51 with lateral sinus thrombosis in the study by Preter et al. [8] and 1 out of 91 patients with CVT in the VENOPORT cohort [5] developed a dural fistula.

On the other hand, in 1 out of 10 cases reported by Enevoldson and Russell [27], in 3 out of 51 patients with lateral sinus thrombosis included in the series by Preter et al. [8], and in 10 out of 624 in the ISCVT cohort [2] a pre-existing dural fistula was identified.

Neuropsychological and Neuropsychiatric Sequelae

There is little information on the long-term neuropsychological and neuropsychiatric outcome in CVT survivors. Madureira et al. [28] investigated professional status, cognitive performance, depressive symptoms and quality of life in 15 consecutive CVT patients 12 months from onset. Forty-seven percent fully regained their previous occupation, 33% changed to part-time work, while 20% retired. Only 2 patients demonstrated neuropsychological impairment. Both had a low score on the Mini-Mental State Examination. One of them was aphasic and the other had verbal memory and verbal fluency impairment. Twenty-seven percent scored >12 points in the Hamilton Depression Rating Scale. Concerning quality of life, as measured by the Euroquol, half of the survivors of CVT complained of pain and 2/3 felt anxious or depressed, despite the apparent general health good recovery (87% of the sample) (fig. 2). Buccino et al. [29] studied 34

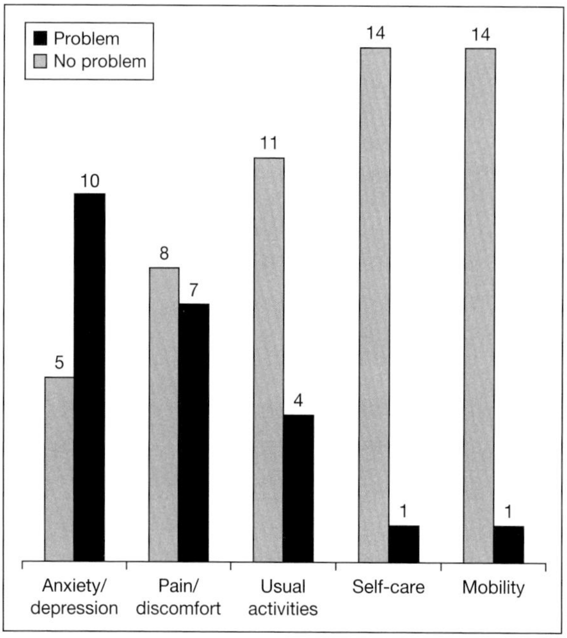

Fig. 2. Quality of life (Euroquol) in dural sinus thrombosis survivors [28].

CVT patients at least 1 year after the acute event (median 3.5 years) and found only 3 cases of mild nonfluent aphasia, working memory deficits in 6 patients and depression of mood in 6 subjects. De Bruijn et al. [30] studied functional outcome, cognitive performance and change in employment status in 59 patients 1 year or more after enrolment in the Dutch-European CVT trial. Twenty percent scored below the 10th percentile in the memory domain, 28% in language, 28% in constructional ability and 33% in visual/spatial orientation/planning. Forty percent could not resume their previous level of economic activity. The discrepancies between de Bruijn et al. [30] and the other two series may be partly explained by the Dutch series being biased towards more severe cases.

Abulia, executive deficits and amnesia, may result from thrombosis of the deep venous system, causing bilateral panthalamic infarcts. Recovery is variable, but memory deficits, behavioral problems or executive deficits may persist [31, 32].

Aphasia, in general of the fluent type, results from left lateral sinus thrombosis with temporal infarct or hemorrhage. Recovery is usually favorable but minor troubles in spontaneous speech and naming may pose important limitations in social interaction and in performing service or intellectual jobs.

Table 2. Outcome of pregnancy after dural sinus thrombosis (CVT)

Study	Women	Pregnancies/ women	Birth	Abortion	CVT/DVT
Srinivasan [33]	135	5/5	5	–	none
Preter et al. [8]	47	16/9	12	4	none
Lamy et al. [34]	68	44/29	26	16	0 CVT
VENOPORT [5]	101	2/2	2	–	none
Mehraein et al. [35]	39	22/14	19	3	none
ISCVT [2]	465	34/24	25	9	1 + 2
Total	855	101/83	89	32	1 + 2

Patients should be reassured about the very low of risk of recurrence of CVT and encouraged to return to previous occupations and hobbies. In some cases antidepressants may be needed.

Future Pregnancies

Pregnancy and in particular puerperium are known risk factors for CVT. Six studies investigated the outcome and complications of pregnancy in women who suffered CVT [2, 8, 5, 33–35], with a total of 855 women under observation, of whom 83 became pregnant (101 pregnancies) after their CVT (table 2). These studies found that the risk of complications during future pregnancies was low. In fact, 88% of the pregnancies ended in a normal birth, the remaining being prematurely terminated by voluntary or by spontaneous abortion. There were only 1 case of recurrent CVT and 2 cases of deep venous thrombosis. A high proportion of spontaneous abortion was, however, noticed.

Based on the available evidence, CVT is not a contraindication for future pregnancies. The same applies for pregnancy/puerperium-related CVT. Antithrombotic prophylaxis during pregnancy is probably unnecessary, unless a prothrombotic condition or a previous thromboembolism has been identified.

References

1 Bousser MG, Ferro JM: Cerebral venous thrombosis: an update. Lancet Neurol 2007;6:162–170.

2 Ferro JM, Canhão P, Stam J, Bousser MG, Barinagarrementeria F; ISCVT Investigators: Prognosis of cerebral vein and dural sinus thrombosis: results of the International Study on Cerebral Vein and Dural Sinus Thrombosis (ISCVT). Stroke 2004;35:664–670.

3 Rondepierre P, Hamon M, Leys D, Lederc X, Mournier-Vehrer F, Godefroy O, Janssens E, Pruvo JP: Thromboses veineuses cérébrales: étude de l'évolution. Rev Neurol 1995;151:100–104.
4 de Bruijn SFTM, de Haan RJ, Stam J; for the Cerebral Venous Sinus Thrombosis Study Group: Clinical features and prognostic factors of cerebral venous sinus thrombosis in a prospective series of 59 patients. J Neurol Neurosurg Psychiatry 2001;70:105–108.
5 Ferro JM, Lopes MG, Rosas MJ, Ferro MA, Fontes J; Cerebral Venous Thrombosis Portuguese Collaborative Study Group (VENOPORT): Long-term prognosis of cerebral vein and dural sinus thrombosis: results of the VENOPORT Study. Cerebrovasc Dis 2002;13:272–278.
6 Breteau G, Mounier-Vehier F, Godefroy O, Gauvrit JY, Mackowiak-Cordoliani MA, Girot M, Bertheloot D, Henon H, Lucas C, Leclerc X, Fourrier F, Pruvo JP, Leys D: Cerebral venous thrombosis: 3-year clinical outcome in 55 consecutive patients. J Neurol 2003;250:29–35.
7 Cakmak S, Derex L, Berruyer M, Nighoghossian N, Philippeau F, Adeleine P, Hermier M, Froment JC, Trouillas P: Cerebral venous thrombosis: clinical outcome and systematic screening of prothrombotic factors. Neurology 2003;60:1175–1178.
8 Preter M, Tzourio CH, Ameri A, Bousser MG: Long term prognosis in cerebral venous thrombosis: a follow-up of 77 patients. Stroke 1996;27:243–246.
9 Gosk-Bierska I, Wysokinski W, Brown RD Jr, Karnicki K, Grill D, Wiste H, Wysokinska E, McBane II RD: Cerebral venous sinus thrombosis. Incidence of venous thrombosis recurrence and survival. Neurology 2006;67:814–819.
10 Baumgartner RW, Studer A, Arnold M, Georgiadis D: Recanalisation of cerebral venous thrombosis. J Neurol Neurosurg Psychiatry 2003;74:459–461.
11 Masuhr F, Mehraein S, Einhäupl K: Cerebral venous and sinus thrombosis. J Neurol 2004;251: 11–23.
12 Maqueda VM, Thijs V: Risk of thromboembolism after cerebral venous thrombosis. Eur J Neurol 2006;13:302–305.
13 Stolz E, Trittmacher S, Rahimi A, Gerriets T, Rottger C, Siekmann R, Kaps M: Influence of recanalization on outcome in dural sinus thrombosis: a prospective study. Stroke 2004;35:544–547.
14 Favrole P, Guichard JP, Crassard I, Bousser MG, Chabriat H: Diffusion-weighted imaging of intravascular clots in cerebral venous thrombosis. Stroke 2004;35:99–103.
15 Strupp M, Covi M, Seelos K, Dichgans M, Brandt T: Cerebral venous thrombosis: correlation between recanalization and clinical outcome – a long-term follow-up of 40 patients. J Neurol 2002;249:1123–1124.
16 Einhäupl K, Bousser MG, de Bruijn SF, Ferro JM, Martinelli I, Masuhr F, Stam J: EFNS guideline on the treatment of cerebral venous and sinus thrombosis. Eur J Neurol 2006;13:553–559.
17 Büller HR, Agnelli G, Hull RH, Hyers TM, Prins MH, Raskob GE: Antithrombotic therapy for venous thromboembolic and thrombolytic therapy. Chest 2004;126:401S–428S.
18 Canhão P, Ferro JM, Bousser M-G, Barinagarrementeria F, Stam J; ISCVT Collaborators: Dural sinus thrombosis presenting as isolated intracranial hypertension: always benign? J Neurol 2005;252(suppl 2):II29.
19 Cumurciuc R, Crassard I, Sarov M, Valade D, Bousser MG: Headache as the only neurological sign of cerebral venous thrombosis: a series of 17 cases. J Neurol Neurosurg Psychiatry 2005;76: 1084–1087.
20 Commission on Epidemiology and Prognosis, International League against Epilepsy. Guidelines for epidemiological studies on epilepsy. Epilepsia 1993;34:592–596.
21 Ferro JM, Correia M, Rosas MJ, Pinto AN, Neves G; Cerebral Venous Thrombosis Portuguese Collaborative Study Group [Venoport]: Seizures in cerebral vein and dural sinus thrombosis. Cerebrovasc Dis 2003;15:78–83.
22 Ferro JM, Canhão P, Bousser MG, Stam J, Barinagarrementeria F; ISCVT Investigators: Early seizures in acute cerebral vein and dural sinus thrombosis (CVT). Prevalence, risk of early recurrence and associated conditions. Cerebrovasc Dis 2006;21(suppl 4):39.
23 Ferro JM, Vasconcelos J, Canhão P, Bousser MG, Stam J, Barinagarrementeria F; ISCVT Investigators: Remote seizures in acute cerebral vein and dural sinus thrombosis (CVT). Incidence and associated conditions. Cerebrovasc Dis 2007;23(suppl 2):48.
24 Biousse V, Ameri A, Bousser M-G: Isolated intracranial hypertension as the only sign of cerebral venous thrombosis. Neurology 1999;53:1537–1542.

25 Bousser MG, Russell RR: Cerebral venous thrombosis; in Warlow CP, Van Gijn J (eds): Major Problems in Neurology. London, WB Saunders, 1997, vol 33, pp 27–29.
26 Phatouros CC, Halbach VV, Dowd CF, Lempert TE, Malek AM, Meyers PM, Higashida RT: Acquired pial arteriovenous fistula following cerebral vein thrombosis. Stroke 1999;30: 2487–2490.
27 Enevoldson TP, Russell RW: Cerebral venous thrombosis. New causes for an old syndrome. Q J Med 1990;77:1255–1275.
28 Madureira S, Canhão P, Ferro JM: Cognitive and behavioural outcome of patients with cerebral venous thrombosis. Cerebrovasc Dis 2001;11(suppl 4):108.
29 Buccino G, Scoditti U, Patteri I, Bertolino, Mancia D: Neurological and cognitive long- term outcome in patients with cerebral vein thrombosis. Acta Neurol Scand 2003;107:330–335.
30 de Bruijn SF, Budde M, Teunisse S, de Haan RJ, Stam J: Long-term outcome of cognition and functional health after cerebral venous sinus thrombosis. Neurology 2000;54:1687–1689.
31 Rousseaux M, Cabaret M, Bernati T, Pruvo JP, Steinling M: Residual deficit of verbal recall after a left internal cerebral vein infarct. Rev Neurol (Paris) 1998;154:401–407.
32 Vucic S, Mackenzie RA: Neuropsychological manifestations in a case of bilateral thalamic infarction. J Clin Neurosci 2003;10:238–242.
33 Srinivasan K: Cerebral venous and arterial thrombosis in pregnancy and puerperium. A study of 135 patients. Angiology 1983;34:731–746.
34 Lamy C, Hamon JB, Coste J, Mas JL: Ischemic stroke in young women: risk of recurrence during subsequent pregnancies. French Study Group on Stroke in Pregnancy. Neurology 2000;55:269–274.
35 Mehraein S, Ortwein H, Busch M, Weih M, Einhäupl K, Masuhr F: Risk of recurrence of cerebral venous and sinus thrombosis during subsequent pregnancy and puerperium. J Neurol Neurosurg Psychiatry 2003;74:814–816.

Prof. José M. Ferro
Department of Neurology, Hospital de Santa Maria
Av. Prof. Egas Moniz
PT–1649-035 Lisboa (Portugal)
Tel./Fax +351 21 7957 474, E-Mail jmferro@fm.ul.pt

Caso V, Agnelli G, Paciaroni M (eds): Handbook on Cerebral Venous Thrombosis.
Front Neurol Neurosci. Basel, Karger, 2008, vol 23, pp 172–178

Long-Term Prognosis of Cerebral Vein and Sinus Thrombosis

Arne Lindgren

Department of Clinical Sciences Lund, Neurology, Lund University, Lund, Sweden

Abstract

In recent reports, cerebral vein and sinus thrombosis has had a better long-term prognosis than previously thought. However, there may be long-term problems that have not attracted enough attention. The aim of this chapter is to examine the literature for studies reporting long-term prognosis and outcome after cerebral vein and sinus thrombosis. The long-term prognosis after cerebral vein and sinus thrombosis mainly depends on underlying diseases, e.g. cancer. If no serious underlying disease is present, the long-term prognosis is generally good. However, death, impaired functional outcome, headache, epileptic seizures, cognitive impairment and recurrent thrombosis occur in some patients. Although the general long-term prognosis after cerebral vein and sinus thrombosis is good, the practicing clinician handling these patients should be aware of certain complications that are not uncommon. Follow-up of these patients is important, even if they initially seem to have recovered completely.

Copyright © 2008 S. Karger AG, Basel

In recent reports, cerebral vein and sinus thrombosis (CVT) has had a better prognosis than previously thought [1, 2]. However, there are several threats for the patients who have suffered from a CVT (table 1). The underlying disease may be serious and this may in itself cause death or impairment for the patient. There is a risk of recurrence of a new venous thrombotic event. There is also the risk of permanent neurological deficits due to parenchymatous lesions associated with the initial thrombosis. Increased intracranial pressure and the thrombosis may lead to compromised venous flow and impaired circulation of cerebrospinal fluid (CSF). Cognitive function impairment may have been underestimated in the past with biased focus on the modified Rankin Scale (mRS) and insufficient assessment of neuropsychological function. The natural history of cerebral vein thrombosis has recently been reviewed [3], as well as prognostic indicators in CVT [4]. This chapter focuses on these questions from

Table 1. Problems that patients may develop during long-term follow-up of CVT

Problem	Proportion[1], %	Comment
Death	1.5[2]	Related to cancer and focal deficit at onset
New thrombotic events	13[3]	Both CVT and DVT may occur
Epileptic seizures	5–16	Almost only among patients with seizures in acute phase
Focal neurological deficits	12–18	Paresis, visual impairment and other
Headache	0–60	Probably rather common after CVT
Incomplete recanalization	6–59	Additional recanalization uncommon after first 3–6 months after CVT onset
Compromised CSF hydrodynamics	100	One study, clinical significance unknown at present
Dural arteriovenous fistulas	1–3	May develop simultaneously or later in relation to CVT
Cognitive impairment	17–35	Higher proportions in studies with detailed examination

CVT = Cerebral vein and sinus thrombosis; DVT = deep vein thrombosis other than cerebral.

[1]After approximately 1 year or more (deaths, focal deficits, etc. only during acute phase not included).

[2]Between 6 and 16 months after onset of CVT.

[3]Also includes events within 1 year after onset of CVT.

a long-term prognostic perspective. In this chapter, long-term is defined as 1 year or more after diagnosis of CVT.

Survival

Even though it was previously thought that CVT was often leading to death, it was suggested already in 1953 that without additional morbid factors, many patients with intracranial venous thrombosis may be capable of recovery [2]. There are several studies of long-term survival after CVT (table 2). However, only four of these studies contain more than 100 patients, and the International Study on Cerebral Vein and Dural Sinus Thrombosis (ISCVT) is by far the largest study [5]. The majority of deaths after CVT occur during the first days and months after onset of the disease [5–7]. In the ISCVT, 4.3% were

Table 2. Studies with at least 20 patients regarding long-term survival after CVT

Study	Patients	Median follow-up	Survival rate, %
Appenzeller et al. [13]	24	46 months[1]	100
Baumgartner et al. [14]	33	12 months	100
Breteau et al. [8]	55	36 months	87
Buccino et al. [10]	38	3.5 years	97
de Bruijn et al. [21]	57	18 months	86
Ferro et al. [6]	142	22 months[1]	92
Ferro et al. [5]	624	16 months	92
Gosk-Bierska [15]	154	36 months[1]	92
Mehraein et al. [16]	115	10.2 years	74
Preter et al. [7]	77	63 months	100[2]
Stolz et al. [11]	79	31 months	82

[1]Indicates mean instead of median value.
[2]Deaths during acute phase not included.

dead at discharge, 6.8% after 6 months and 8.3% at last follow-up (which took place after a median of 16 months in that report) [5]. Death after the acute phase may often be caused by underlying serious disease, e.g. cancer [8]. Focal deficits and cancer in the acute phase are independent predictors of dependence or death at 3 years [8]. However, even though most patients with CVT survive, no less than 3/4 of these survivors have been reported to have some residual symptoms [8]. The prognosis after CVT during pregnancy and puerperium is probably better than after CVT from other causes [4]. Information about CVT in children is scarce but in one study, only 1 of 13 surviving children with CVT died between 1 and 3 years after onset and this death was related to cancer [9]. In summary, if the patient survives during the first months after CVT onset, the risk of subsequent death is small.

Functional Outcome

The survivors after CVT often have a good functional outcome when assessed with the mRS [10]. In the large ISCVT study, at a median follow-up of 16 months, no less than 79% of the initial 624 patients had an mRS of 0 or 1, indicating no or only minor residual symptoms [5]. Multivariate predictors of dependence (mRS 3–5) or death at follow-up were: age above 37 years, male sex, coma, mental status disorder, hemorrhage on admission CT scan, thrombosis of the deep cerebral venous system, CNS infection and cancer [5]. Stolz et al. [11] found that 50 of 56 (89%) survivors after a median follow-up of 31 months had an mRS score of 0 or 1. Buccino et al. [10] reported that none of their 34 surviving patients examined at a median of 3.5 years after CVT onset had functional disability when examined with the mRS. However, in spite of this, several of their patients had cognitive problems or indications of depression [10]. Although the prognosis may be more serious after thrombosis of the deep cerebral venous system [5], even patients with isolated deep cerebral venous thrombosis with decreased consciousness may sometimes have an excellent outcome [12].

Permanent Neurological Deficits and Headache

Focal neurological deficit has been reported in 12–18% of patients at long-term follow-up after CVT [8, 13, 14]. This includes motor deficits, visual field defects and aphasia [8, 14]. Visual field defects have been observed in 10% of survivors [8]. Permanent optic atrophy may be present because of increased intracranial pressure in the acute phase and cause impaired vision [7]. In several reports, headache is also a common problem after CVT and has been reported in 25% [13] and up to 60% of survivors [8], although much lower proportions have also been reported [14].

Epileptic Seizures

Epileptic seizures are not uncommon after the acute phase of CVT and have been reported in 5–16% of long-term survivors [4, 7, 11]. Epileptic seizures in the chronic phase after CVT mainly occur among patients who already had seizures in the acute phase [4]. Therefore, antiepileptic drug therapy can in the first place be reserved for patients with seizures during the acute phase of CVT [see the chapter by Ferro and Canhão, this vol., pp. 161–171].

New Thrombotic Events

It has been reported that the risk of recurrent venous thrombotic events for patients with CVT is similar to that of patients with lower extremity deep vein thrombosis (DVT) [15]. In this study, the proportion of CVT patients with a recurrent cerebral venous thrombosis was 6.5% after a mean follow-up of 36 months [15]. However, the recurrent venous thrombosis in CVT patients may not only occur in the cerebral venous system but also in other locations, e.g. in the lower extremities. Most recurrences seem to occur within the 1st year [7, 15]. In one study of 154 patients, the authors did not find variables significantly associated with recurrent venous thrombosis in their patients [15] [see the chapter by Ferro and Canhão, this vol., pp. 161–171].

The risk of recurrent CVT during subsequent pregnancy and puerperium seems to be very low [7]. In one study of 39 women with initial sinus thrombosis during childbearing age, during a mean follow-up of 10 years, the authors observed 22 pregnancies in 14 women without recurrence of CVT or DVT [16]. In the ISCVT study, only one CVT and two DVTs were observed during subsequent pregnancies in 34 women [5]. The teratogenic risk of warfarin has to be borne in mind, and if anticoagulation treatment is indicated during pregnancy, treatment with low-molecular heparin drugs should instead be considered [see the chapter by Ferro and Canhão, this vol., pp. 163–171].

Dural Arteriovenous Fistulas

CVT has been reported in 39% of patients with dural arteriovenous fistulas (DAFs) [17]. CVT and DAFs may develop simultaneously in the acute phase in the same patient or DAFs may develop later after a CVT. One possible reason for the association between CVT and DAFs is that the increased venous pressure in CVT may cause an opening of the arteriovenous shunts between meningeal arteries and the dural venous sinuses with a subsequent development of a fistule [17]. The proportion of CVT patients that develop DAFs is probably low [7, 11] but a DAF should be considered if a patient with CVT has signs of hemorrhage or infarct in the brain parenchyma, seizures or altered mental status. MR imaging and MR angiography may be used to assess DAFs [18] [see the chapter by Ferro and Canhão, this vol., pp. 161–171].

Recanalization and Impaired CSF Circulation

Recanalization of the thrombosed cerebral venous system seems to mostly occur during the first 4 months after CVT onset but to be rare thereafter [14]. The superior sagittal sinus had the highest rate of recanalization (94%) and the sigmoid sinus the lowest (41%) in one study [14]. In one study, recanalization did not influence outcome at 12 months, and it was suggested that frequent examinations to determine recanalization may not be useful to determine patient outcome [19]. It has been shown that patients with previous superior sagittal sinus thrombosis may have compromised CSF hydrodynamics during a long time after the acute phase of CVT [20]. Kristensen et al. [20] showed that all of their 10 patients examined after a mean of 5.8 years after superior sagittal sinus thrombosis had such changes with persistently raised CSF pressure mainly due to raised pressure in the sagittal sinus, even though a clinical impact of this was not observed [20]. The authors suggested that the changed CSF hydrodynamics was probably most often caused by increased CSF pressure rather than obstructed resorption of CSF [20].

Cognitive Impairment

Even though the survival rate is good and most patients with CVT have no or only minor dependency when assessed with the mRS, there seems to be a considerable proportion of patients with cognitive impairment following CVT. In a more detailed examination of cognitive function after CVT, de Bruijn et al. [21] reported that 35% of their patients had cognitive impairment and that 40% had symptoms leading to restrictions in lifestyle when assessed after a mean time of 18.5 months after inclusion in their study. Another study reported cognitive dysfunction in 17% of the patients after a mean follow-up of 46 months [13]. Deficits in working memory and depression may also occur after CVT [10]. The 'hidden' complication of cognitive impairment is probably at risk of being greatly underestimated with the mRS examination. Therefore, cognitive function has to be specifically assessed in all patients after a CVT [see the chapter by Ferro and Canhão, this vol., pp. 161–171].

Conclusions

The long-term prognosis after cerebral vein and sinus thrombosis is generally very good. The survival rate after the acute phase of CVT has been passed is high but some patients encounter remaining problems. These include focal neurological deficits, headache, epileptic seizures, cognitive impairment and depression. It is therefore important to follow up these patients even if they initially seem to have recovered completely.

References

1 Nagpal RD: Dural sinus and cerebral venous thrombosis. Neurosurg Rev 1983;6:155–160.
2 Barnett HJ, Hyland HH: Noninfective intracranial venous thrombosis. Brain 1953;76:36–49.
3 Dentali F, Gianni M, Crowther MA, Ageno W: Natural history of cerebral vein thrombosis: a systematic review. Blood 2006;108:1129–1134.
4 Hameed B, Syed NA: Prognostic indicators in cerebral venous sinus thrombosis. J Pak Med Assoc 2006;56:551–554.

5 Ferro JM, Canhao P, Stam J, Bousser MG, Barinagarrementeria F: Prognosis of cerebral vein and dural sinus thrombosis: results of the International Study on Cerebral Vein and Dural Sinus Thrombosis (ISCVT). Stroke 2004;35:664–670.
6 Ferro JM, Lopes MG, Rosas MJ, Ferro MA, Fontes J: Long-term prognosis of cerebral vein and dural sinus thrombosis. Results of the VENOPORT study. Cerebrovasc Dis 2002;13:272–278.
7 Preter M, Tzourio C, Ameri A, Bousser MG: Long-term prognosis in cerebral venous thrombosis. Follow-up of 77 patients. Stroke 1996;27:243–246.
8 Breteau G, Mounier-Vehier F, Godefroy O, Gauvrit JY, Mackowiak-Cordoliani MA, Girot M, Bertheloot D, Henon H, Lucas C, Leclerc X, Fourrier F, Pruvo JP, Leys D: Cerebral venous thrombosis 3-year clinical outcome in 55 consecutive patients. J Neurol 2003;250:29–35.
9 De Schryver EL, Blom I, Braun KP, Kappelle LJ, Rinkel GJ, Peters AC, Jennekens-Schinkel A: Long-term prognosis of cerebral venous sinus thrombosis in childhood. Dev Med Child Neurol 2004;46:514–519.
10 Buccino G, Scoditti U, Patteri I, Bertolino C, Mancia D: Neurological and cognitive long-term outcome in patients with cerebral venous sinus thrombosis. Acta Neurol Scand 2003;107:330–335.
11 Stolz E, Rahimi A, Gerriets T, Kraus J, Kaps M: Cerebral venous thrombosis: an all or nothing disease? Prognostic factors and long-term outcome. Clin Neurol Neurosurg 2005;107:99–107.
12 Kamal AK, Itrat A, Shoukat S, Khealani A, Kamal K: Isolated deep venous thrombosis – case series, literature review and long term follow-up. J Pak Med Assoc 2006;56:557–559.
13 Appenzeller S, Zeller CB, Annichino-Bizzachi JM, Costallat LT, Deus-Silva L, Voetsch B, Faria AV, Zanardi VA, Damasceno BP, Cendes F: Cerebral venous thrombosis: influence of risk factors and imaging findings on prognosis. Clin Neurol Neurosurg 2005;107:371–378.
14 Baumgartner RW, Studer A, Arnold M, Georgiadis D: Recanalisation of cerebral venous thrombosis. J Neurol Neurosurg Psychiatry 2003;74:459–461.
15 Gosk-Bierska I, Wysokinski W, Brown RD Jr, Karnicki K, Grill D, Wiste H, Wysokinska E, McBane RD 2nd: Cerebral venous sinus thrombosis: incidence of venous thrombosis recurrence and survival. Neurology 2006;67:814–819.
16 Mehraein S, Ortwein H, Busch M, Weih M, Einhaupl K, Masuhr F: Risk of recurrence of cerebral venous and sinus thrombosis during subsequent pregnancy and puerperium. J Neurol Neurosurg Psychiatry 2003;74:814–816.
17 Tsai LK, Jeng JS, Liu HM, Wang HJ, Yip PK: Intracranial dural arteriovenous fistulas with or without cerebral sinus thrombosis: analysis of 69 patients. J Neurol Neurosurg Psychiatry 2004;75:1639–1641.
18 Kwon BJ, Han MH, Kang HS, Chang KH: MR imaging findings of intracranial dural arteriovenous fistulas: relations with venous drainage patterns. AJNR Am J Neuroradiol 2005;26:2500–2507.
19 Stolz E, Trittmacher S, Rahimi A, Gerriets T, Rottger C, Siekmann R, Kaps M: Influence of recanalization on outcome in dural sinus thrombosis: a prospective study. Stroke 2004;35:544–547.
20 Kristensen B, Malm J, Markgren P, Ekstedt J: CSF hydrodynamics in superior sagittal sinus thrombosis. J Neurol Neurosurg Psychiatry 1992;55:287–293.
21 de Bruijn SF, Budde M, Teunisse S, de Haan RJ, Stam J: Long-term outcome of cognition and functional health after cerebral venous sinus thrombosis. Neurology 2000;54:1687–1689.

Arne Lindgren, MD, PhD, Associate Professor
Department of Clinical Sciences Lund, Neurology, Lund University
SE–221 85 Lund (Sweden)
Tel. +46 46171424, Fax +46 46158919, E-Mail arne.lindgren@med.lu.se

Author Index

Subject Index